The Health Collection

provided by

Genesis Health Services

Foundation

DIET FOR THE
MIND

DIET FOR THE
MIND

*The Latest Science on
What to Eat to Prevent Alzheimer's and
Cognitive Decline — from the Creator
of the MIND Diet*

Dr. Martha Clare Morris

WITH 80 RECIPES BY LAURA MORRIS

LITTLE, BROWN AND COMPANY
New York   Boston   London

Little, Brown and Company
Hachette Book Group
1290 Avenue of the Americas, New York, NY 10104
littlebrown.com

First Edition: December 2017

Little, Brown and Company is a division of Hachette Book Group, Inc. The Little, Brown name and logo are trademarks of Hachette Book Group, Inc.

The Hachette Speakers Bureau provides a wide range of authors for speaking events. To find out more, go to hachettespeakersbureau.com or call (866) 376-6591.

Interior photography by Kristen Mendiola, styled by Sherrie Tan

ISBN 978-0-316-44115-5

LCCN 2017952226

10 9 8 7 6 5 4 3 2 1

LSC-C

Printed in the United States

In Loving Memory of
James Joseph Morris, Jr.
A spirit who consumed food
and all that life has to offer with gusto

Contents

Contents

Introduction:
Where the Heart and Mind
Meet

I believe that some of the best contributions to the greater good begin with our passions—and this book is no different. In 2009, my daughter Laura and I began planning what would eventually become *Diet for the MIND*. At the time, Laura was a certified personal trainer and nutrition consultant, about to begin her training at the Northwest Culinary Academy of Vancouver. She wanted to build on her already formidable skills in creating meals that were both delicious and nutritious. Simultaneously, I was establishing a new academic program in nutrition at Rush University in Chicago called "Nutritional Medicine." The program was designed to teach practicing medical professionals—doctors, nurses, pharmacists, dentists, physical therapists, and the like—about the influence of nutrition on health and disease. Unfortunately, nutrition education is barely a footnote in medical training programs, yet it's at the core of all matters in health and disease. This program was an attempt to bridge the gap in US medical education.

As part of the Nutritional Medicine program, I invited the leading experts in nutrition science to Chicago to lecture on different diseases. The courses were designed to take place in a two-day seminar series, three times a year. For each seminar, we flew in three or four distinguished guest lecturers from all over the country. Because of my doctoral training in nutritional epidemiology at the Harvard School of Public Health (recently renamed the Harvard T.H. Chan School of Public Health), I was fortunate to have many mentors and college friends who were the "best of the best" with respect to nutrition and health. Among these famous guest lecturers were faculty of Harvard University and the Harvard studies on nutrition and health, including Walter Willett, Frank Sacks, JoAnn Manson, Michelle Williams, Eric Rimm, Susan Hankinson, and Alberto Ascherio; and faculty of the Friedman School of Nutrition Science and Policy at Tufts University, including Irwin Rosenberg, Katherine Tucker, and Sarah Booth.

For each seminar, we invited all the lecturers to my home for a cozy gathering around a brain-healthy dinner. Laura created and prepared the meals, and each course was paired with a different craft beer created by my son-in-law Peter Crowley (husband of my older daughter, Clare), an international award-winning brewmaster and owner of Haymarket Pub & Brewery. Laura and I had many discussions around the planning of the meal courses so that they merged her dazzling skills with what we know about the science of nutrition and the brain. Once the meal plan was set, we enlisted Pete to pair each course with one of his craft beers to enhance the flavors and essence of the culinary experience.

As each dinner course was served, Laura and other members of our family described the food and beer contents, and their pairing flavors. We had such fun planning and executing these dinners, and our guests enjoyed the amazing talents of Chef Laura and Beer Maestro Pete. However, the star of these dinners, so lovingly prepared and delivered in honor of our celebrated guests, was my late husband, Jim. Jim had been diagnosed with head and neck cancer in February 2008. He was unable to eat or drink by mouth very early on in his four-and-a-half-year battle with the disease, and by 2011, he was barely able to talk. Despite his inability to enjoy the feast and participate in the lively conversation, Jim — the ultimate master of hospitality — participated in one of his favorite activities by assisting Laura as sous chef and serving each dinner course to the guests. Jim died in May 2012 and was not able to be part of the program's later dinners. Other family members stepped in to help, including my sister-in-law Louise and future daughter-in-law Rachel.

The discussions Laura and I had around the planning and preparation of these dinners were the seeds for this book. It is the culmination of our mutual passion for nutrition and health and, most of all, for the love of family and friends. Food is central to the expression of love. My passion for nutrition arose with my first pregnancy and grew with my desire to ensure that my children were as healthy as they could possibly be. My other passion is science, and I was able to marry the two during my doctoral training in nutritional epidemiology at the Harvard School of Public Health.

For the past twenty years, I have been at the forefront of research in an area with tremendous implications for public health: the link between Alzheimer's disease, cognitive decline, and diet. In 2015 my team put all this research together to develop the MIND diet score, which we found was associated with reduced risk of Alzheimer's disease and slower cognitive decline. It is this research that I describe in part I of the book. I am eager to share what I've learned about this cutting-edge science as well as to share nutritious, easy-to-prepare recipes that support it. The eighty selections in part II of this book were created by Laura, who not only trained at a renowned culinary institute, but also grew up in a home where cooking and family meals were treasured and good nutrition was emphasized. Many of these recipes are family favorites for casual dinners or special occasions. They're quick and easy to make, budget friendly, and ideal for everyday living. Both delicious and satisfying, the meals can also be used as a template for daily or weekly food plans or, if you are an experienced cook, as a healthy base for your own dishes. Laura and I hope you will enjoy them while also reaping the benefits they're bound to create.

Jim's love of food, family, and the camaraderie of meals and conversation is a fond memory and an important foundation of our children's upbringing. The Morris family table is famous for good food and conversation. We've shared our table with many guests, and Jim was always a central part of these meals. This book is dedicated to him. He endeavored to enjoy every second of his sixty-six years of life, and he made everyone around him enjoy life, too.

PART I

MIND-HEALTHY SCIENCE

CHAPTER 1

Cognitive Decline and Dementia

As we age, our brains age, too. Our ability to think slows down, and we may experience occasional difficulty in, for example, recalling where we left our keys or retrieving a word or name. By all accounts, this is considered a normal degree of cognitive decline. It is a very different and more painful story, however, when you can no longer remember the way to get home or the names of your grandchildren. That is the experience of those who suffer from dementia, including Alzheimer's disease. No wonder dementia and cognitive decline are among the most feared consequences of aging. Being able to reason, remember, and make decisions the way we always have connects us to the identity, personality traits, and relationships we spend our lives building. To live out our golden years with a healthy degree of brainpower is what we all hope for our future. I am happy to say that there is a great deal we can do to make this the reality for much of our lifetime.

Dementia is a widespread and growing public health problem. In 2015, Alzheimer's disease, the leading type of dementia, affected more than five million adults in the United States and was the sixth leading cause of death. And while Alzheimer's disease accounts for some 60 to 80 percent of all cases of dementia, many adults experience other forms of dementia, with symptoms including memory loss, difficulties with communication and language, trouble with focus and attention, and errors in visual perception, reasoning, and judgment. Fully one in three seniors dies with Alzheimer's or another form of dementia. At this time, there is no cure for Alzheimer's disease, and the treatments are largely ineffective. But take heart: the picture for prevention is not as bleak as we once thought.

At one time, Alzheimer's disease was thought to be genetic, and the signs of dementia, like memory loss and confusion, were thought to be inevitable consequences of aging. However, over the last thirty to forty years, researchers have identified many factors that can cause or prevent the disease, most of which can be managed with effective treatments and/or through healthy lifestyle choices. This means that it is possible to delay the symptoms of dementia in later life by taking control of your health in your young and middle-aged adult years. And because many of these factors are known to be important for heart health, by adopting healthy lifestyle choices, you will be increasing your chances of maintaining not only a healthy brain but a healthy heart, too.

Rest assured that debilitating cognitive decline does not have to be your destiny. In fact, in this book you will learn many ways to keep your brain functioning at its best and your overall health vibrant as you age—and a lot of this has to do with what is on your plate. I am often asked whether young or middle-aged adults need to be concerned with changing their diet to prevent Alzheimer's disease or to keep their brain healthy in old age, and the answer is a resounding yes! Key studies that followed young adult populations into old age observed that high levels of blood pressure, blood cholesterol, and obesity in middle age were associated with increased risk of developing Alzheimer's disease and other dementias in old age. Healthy behaviors over a lifetime do matter, in terms of both optimum functioning in the moment and your health in the future. It is never too early or too late, and you are never too old to benefit from a healthy diet and lifestyle that preserve your mind and overall health.

In this chapter, I'll describe the difference between normal cognitive aging and dementia, as well as the primary risk factors for dementia and why diet is important. I'll discuss the role that supportive organs, like the heart, play in mind preservation and how oxidative stress and inflammation fit into the picture. Throughout, I have taken a strong scientific approach that encompasses the highest-quality data out there. My diet suggestions are based on a thorough review of the scientific literature from a broad spectrum of animal and human investigations — not just my own research. Each nutrient and food that I propose for brain health has the foundational backing of demonstrated biological mechanisms in the brain, metabolic system, or cardiovascular system and consistent results among high-quality epidemiological studies to support its relationship with health in human populations. In other words, every food and nutrient proposed is based on scientific evidence.

As a researcher, scientific evidence is obviously important to me, but it should also be important to you when creating a nutrition plan that supports your mind and body. If you're being asked to tweak your diet, you deserve a substantial set of reasons why. Change is hard, and you shouldn't have to cut back on cheese and meat just because I think it's a good idea! Scientific evidence, on the other hand, is obtained through the systematic study of behavior and biological systems. This means that it is not a general impression formed by, say, a medical doctor through the evaluation and treatment of patients. It is also not the extrapolation of biochemical properties of cells in the petri dish to the hugely complex disease state in the human body. There are many ways in which these two theoretical approaches to disease causation are faulty and likely to result in theories that are completely off the mark. Unfortunately, they are the foundation of all too many books on diet and disease. What you will find here is advice based on my comprehensive review of the most rigorous scientific studies of nutrition and the brain. As an epidemiologist, my expertise is on the strengths and weaknesses of research study designs. This has allowed me to filter out the biased and unreliable studies and to focus on the strongest scientific evidence to identify the foods and nutrients that are important to brain health.

WHAT'S DIET GOT TO DO WITH IT?

Following a diet that is based on scientifically driven dietary recommendations is one of the most assured ways to keep your brain functioning at its best. You may have read that exercising, learning new tasks, and keeping socially active are helpful—and they sure are—but none of these activities would be possible without the right foods to fuel the brain.

The food you eat does more for your body than simply fill your stomach and satisfy your taste buds. At its most basic, you would die without food, because every organ of the body requires nutrients and other dietary components to function. Some of these dietary components are used to form basic cell structures. For example, dietary fats are incorporated into the membranes of neurons, or nerve cells, and the *type* of fat determines how well neurons transmit signals to other nerve cells in the brain or to your muscles and other organs. The omega-3 fatty acid DHA (docosahexaenoic acid), which comes from foods like fish and walnuts, is an important part of a brain-healthy diet. In fact, when DHA is part of the neuron's surrounding membrane, it makes that neuron flexible and dynamic. This improves neurotransmission, which in turn impacts your ability to think more clearly and quickly. Also required are nutrients like folate, which builds DNA and new cells, and the powerful antioxidant vitamin E, which protects cells against oxidative injury. Other dietary components like carbohydrates and fats provide the fuels that are necessary for organs to function, including your brain.

The growing ranks of middle-aged and older adults in the population, along with commonly held fears of losing one's memories and the ability to think, have increased the demand for dietary guidelines. I can speak directly to this demand because the link between Alzheimer's disease, cognitive decline, and diet has been my major focus of research for the past twenty years. I am the principal investigator of the diet studies in two large population-based studies conducted at Rush University of risk factors for the development of Alzheimer's disease, cognitive decline, and other common problems in older people. One of these studies, the Chicago Health and Aging Project (CHAP), began in 1993 and includes more than ten thousand residents age sixty-five and older living on the south side of Chicago. Participants of the study were evaluated every three years for health and lifestyle behaviors. Neurological evaluations for the diagnosis of Alzheimer's disease and other dementias were also performed on a smaller number of randomly selected participants. The second study, the Memory and Aging Project (MAP), includes more than eighteen hundred residents living in retirement communities and senior public housing throughout the Chicago metropolitan area. Participants of the MAP study are evaluated annually for neurological conditions, cognitive abilities, and diet, among many other factors, and all participants have agreed to donate their brains when they die. These studies, funded by multiple grants from the National Institutes of Health and the Alzheimer's Association, have generated numerous findings of dietary associations with neurodegenerative diseases like Alzheimer's and have helped shape my understanding of how diet can affect the way the brain ages and potentially declines. The results of these studies were also instrumental in my team's development of the MIND (Mediterranean-DASH Intervention for Neurodegenerative Delay) diet to prevent cognitive decline and Alzheimer's disease. We are currently conducting a large randomized trial of the MIND diet that will be the definitive test of whether the diet is truly protective against cognitive decline and neurodegenerative changes to the brain.

To briefly sum up the findings of my Rush diet studies, we found that study participants had a lower risk of Alzheimer's disease and slower rate of cognitive decline with:

- An intake of vitamin E in their diet

- Intakes of vitamin B_{12}, folate, and niacin

- Intakes of lutein, beta-carotene, and flavonoids

- Consumption of seafood and omega-3 fatty acids

- Daily consumption of vegetables—in particular, leafy green vegetables

- Dietary fat composition that is low in saturated and trans fats and high in vegetable fats

We'll explore these dietary factors in later chapters, along with recipes that incorporate the foods that best support them.

COGNITIVE AGING 101

Cognitive function—or more simply, your ability to think—is central to navigating everyday life. Reasoning, planning, remembering, using language to communicate, and processing information efficiently are a few ways that you do this. In fact, simply getting dressed in the morning involves many of these cognitive skills all at once. You use reasoning to realize it's cold outside and you should put on wool pants instead of shorts; planning, to first take off your pajamas and underwear before putting on clean clothes; and memory, to remember where you keep your clean clothes. We are not even aware of how much our cognitive skills get us through the day—until, that is, we observe the breakdown of these skills in a person with dementia.

Most of us will experience some decline in thinking abilities as we age as part of the normal aging process. Even so, there is a lot of variability from one person to the next in the rate at which thinking abilities decline, just as there is a lot of variability in peak intelligence. By peak intelligence, I mean our most fully developed intelligence, which occurs at some point in young adulthood. A host of factors determine a person's peak intelligence, including genetics, education, nutrition, and physical activity, to name just a few. Environmental and social factors also play a role—just as good nutrition and lots of exercise contribute to a better functioning brain, a person who grew up in an environment with books, games, and a lot of positive interactions with loving adults will benefit intellectually. And while aspects of these factors will also impact the rate at which your cognitive abilities decline during old age, the degree to which these early life factors affect cognitive decline is not currently known. What we *do* know is that a well-developed and healthy brain going into old age has a far greater capacity to ward off infections, oxidation, and other injuries that are a part of normal life. Biologically speaking, an optimally developed brain is likely to have more neurons and neural connections to carry on brain function when neurons die or cell systems fail, both of which are an inevitable consequence of aging.

In the large Chicago Health and Aging Project population study I mentioned earlier, we measured cognitive abilities of the same individuals every three years. One of the things we did was track how each person's mental function changed over six years, across participants age sixty-five and older—years in which cognitive decline is most likely and apparent. What's interesting is that many people did not exhibit decline over the six-year period, or even improved their scores on the cognitive tests, and the rates of decline for others ranged from a little to quite a bit. Studies that investigate cognitive decline are designed to identify the factors that are associated with either an increase or decrease in individual rates of decline. The best scientific evidence comes from studies that use multiple cognitive tests to measure a range of cognitive abilities and that use multiple time points of cognitive assessment. This type of study design makes it possible to tease apart individuals' peak cognitive performance from the decline in that peak ability. When you consider how complex the brain is, and all the different types of thinking skills that go into everyday activities, you can appreciate that measuring all of this with accuracy is quite difficult but also essential.

The best studies, then, are those that use a number of tests to measure each cognitive skill, such as memory, attention, reasoning, and thinking speed. The use of multiple cognitive tests ensures that researchers have an accurate picture of a person's thinking ability at that point in time. Now, to investigate changes in thinking abilities, we need to conduct these tests multiple times over a number of years. In the Rush Memory and Aging Project, nineteen cognitive tests are administered to the study participants every year, and many of the participants have been in the study for ten years or more. This kind of study provides precise information about cognitive decline. As you can imagine, this is also expensive and time-consuming; for that reason, there are few studies out there with this kind of extensive information on cognitive decline. In fact, many of the studies in the field of aging have used just one test to measure cognitive function, and have administered the test at just one or two points in time. It is difficult to interpret the findings from these kinds of studies, particularly those with just one test at one time point. And in these cases, it is not possible to separate a person's peak intelligence during his or her younger adult years from declines due to aging or disease. That's why long-term assessments are not only the best way for us to understand a disease process but also the most precise way for us to translate what we've learned into advice that will help you live your very best life. The advice that I give in this book is backed up by findings from these high-quality research studies conducted at Rush.

WHEN COGNITIVE DECLINE ISN'T DEMENTIA

Dementia is a general term for decline in mental abilities that is severe enough to interfere with daily life. There are a number of different types of dementia, but the primary ones are Alzheimer's disease, vascular dementia, and Lewy body dementia. They are largely distinguished by the type of pathology found in the brain. Lewy body dementia, for instance, occurs when protein deposits, called Lewy bodies, accumulate in the neurons, which causes them to die. Lewy bodies are also found in patients with Parkinson's disease, which is a progressive disorder of the nervous system that affects movement. There are also dementias associated with nutrient deficiencies, such as pellagra, a disease caused by niacin deficiency, and hypocobalaminemia, a neurologic syndrome caused by vitamin B_{12} deficiency. Alzheimer's disease is the most common type of dementia.

Many older people — some 15 to 20 percent — will experience a significant decline in their usual cognitive abilities, such as memory or reasoning, but not to the extent that it interferes with their ability to perform daily-life activities. This condition is known as mild cognitive impairment (MCI). Individuals who have MCI are still able to take care of their usual responsibilities. Even though they are at increased risk of developing dementia, many people with MCI never present with the disease.

A significant amount of age-related cognitive decline can't be attributed to the brain pathologies that have been identified and associated with dementia. In fact, a number of treatable conditions can cause *dementia-like* symptoms. Some of the more common ones are depression, drug use and interactions, thyroid problems, alcohol abuse, and certain vitamin deficiencies. If you notice problems with your memory or thinking abilities, please see a doctor, preferably a neurologist, who can evaluate you for these conditions.

Thyroid issues and vitamin B_{12} deficiency, for instance, are two of the more common alternative causes for dementia-like symptoms. Hypothyroidism, or low thyroid levels, affects one in eight adults —

with women being more than five times as likely to have this condition than men, and about 60 percent go undiagnosed! Confusion and memory loss are among these symptoms, along with weight gain, low energy, fatigue, depression, and stiffness or aches in muscles and joints. Daily use of the synthetic thyroid hormone levothyroxine restores thyroid levels and reverses the symptoms. And then there's vitamin B_{12} deficiency. A small percentage of vitamin B_{12} deficiency cases are due to a condition called pernicious anemia, caused by an inability to absorb vitamin B_{12}. However, many more middle-aged and older adults have insufficient levels of vitamin B_{12} due to less efficient absorption, common with aging; low intake of vitamin B_{12}–containing foods; excessive alcohol consumption; or use of antacids and other medications that lower the acidity of the stomach, which makes it harder to absorb vitamin B_{12} from the diet. Vitamin B_{12} is essential to the formation and maintenance of myelin, a fatty sheath that covers the axons of neurons and enhances electrical impulses in neurotransmission. This vitamin is obtained almost exclusively from animal products, such as meats, fish, eggs, cheese, and milk — so vegans, vegetarians, or others who consume a limited amount of animal products are at greater risk of insufficient nutrient intake of vitamin B_{12}.

Middle-aged and older adults who experience low levels of energy, shortness of breath, tingling in their fingers, confusion, or depression would do well to have their physicians check whether their levels of vitamin B_{12} are low or low-normal. Depending on the reason for vitamin B_{12} insufficiency, vitamin supplements or monthly injections may be the most effective way to restore the vitamin levels. Without treatment, vitamin B_{12} deficiency syndrome can cause irreversible neurologic damage, including cognitive impairment. Vitamin B_1 (thiamin) and vitamin B_3 (niacin) also have deficiency syndromes that involve cognitive impairment, but deficiencies in these nutrients are rare in the United States, and the scientific evidence to link low-normal dietary intake of these vitamins to cognitive decline or dementia is limited.

A DETAILED LOOK AT ALZHEIMER'S DISEASE

Dementia that entails a decline in memory-related abilities is central to Alzheimer's disease. And while memory loss is the defining clinical characteristic of Alzheimer's, to be diagnosed with the disease, a second type of cognitive impairment must also be evident. Such deterioration could include problems paying attention, orienting to time or place, understanding the lines of a story or conversation, communicating an idea to others, understanding visual images and spatial relationships, or making the right decision when presented with alternative options.

The memory loss that is associated with Alzheimer's disease is much more serious than the mild, occasional mental lapses that come with normal aging—for instance, temporarily forgetting the name of an acquaintance. Alzheimer's disease typically begins in the part of the brain that controls learning, so one of the early symptoms is difficulty remembering newly learned information. In this scenario, the person might have trouble remembering appointments or upcoming events or need to rely more heavily on memory aids like reminder notes. Another early sign is asking for the same information repeatedly. An initial Alzheimer's diagnosis commonly comes when a family member notices that a loved one asks the same questions over and over and also has problems with dressing or preparing a meal, or is suddenly mismanaging money. Think of the sixty-five-year-old man who can't figure out how he's related to his son and doesn't know how to operate a can opener, or the fifty-year-old woman who can no longer manage her checkbook to pay bills and gets lost driving to the local grocery store.

As the disease progresses, those with Alzheimer's lose their ability to carry on a conversation, may be confused about time and place, and are unable to make good decisions. They become easy prey for telemarketers and others who convince them to give out large amounts of money. More severe stages of the disease may result in disorientation; mood and behavior changes; confusion about events, time, and place; baseless suspicions about family, caregivers, or friends; delusions and depression; and difficulty speaking, swallowing, and walking. Eventually, a person with Alzheimer's disease loses the ability to carry out basic daily activities like dressing, bathing, eating, or using the bathroom.

Inside the Alzheimer's Brain

As we age, most of us will have some degree of one or more pathologies — or disease characteristics — in the brain that are linked to different dementias. In fact, it is rare that the brain of an older person has no evidence of brain pathology. The two that are typical of Alzheimer's disease are beta amyloid plaques and neurofibrillary tangles.

Amyloid plaques occur when an abnormal protein called beta amyloid accumulates into a plaque that forms outside of the nerve cells, or neurons. The amyloid plaques can interfere with communication among these cells. Nerve cells make up the brain, the central nervous system of the spinal cord, and the nervous system that extends into our arms, our legs, and our body's organs. These cells are highly electric so they can process and transmit information to other cells through neural networks. When amyloid plaques build up in the brain, they interfere with the neurons' ability to communicate with one another to produce a memory or perform a task.

Neurofibrillary tangles are tangled nerve filaments that occur within the neuron itself, making it difficult for the neuron to function properly. These filaments are like tubes that transport nutrients and other essential molecules within the cell. A protein called tau is an essential component of these nerve filaments. When tau is damaged, it collapses into twisted strands called tangles. Amyloid plaques and neurofibrillary tangles are found in almost every older brain to some degree. It is the *extent* of the neuropathology that determines whether someone is diagnosed with Alzheimer's disease. Plaques and tangles in the brain will lead to neuron loss, and the brain tissue will gradually atrophy. Brain atrophy is substantial in severe stages of Alzheimer's disease. The hippocampus, a primary brain region involved in memory, is one of the first areas where these plaques and tangles begin to form in people who develop Alzheimer's disease.

Very commonly, individuals will have not just one type of disease neuropathology but multiple neuropathologies—for example, some combination of plaques and tangles, brain infarcts (causing strokes), and/or Lewy bodies. In the Rush community studies that followed groups of individuals who initially didn't have dementia all the way to their death, it was discovered that in the brains of participants with neuropathologically defined dementia, more than two-thirds (68 percent) had Alzheimer's disease neuropathology, and more than half had multiple neuropathologic diagnoses.[1] The most common combination was of Alzheimer's disease and stroke— that is, these brains had brain infarcts in addition to Alzheimer's plaques and tangles. It was also discovered that the more types of neuropathologies present in the brain, the greater the chance that the participants showed signs of dementia before their death. Those who had multiple neuropathologic diagnoses were actually three times more likely to exhibit signs of dementia when they were alive.

Recent advances in brain imaging and Alzheimer's disease research have taught us a great deal about the very beginnings of dementia, twenty to thirty years before clinical symptoms occur. The National Institute on Aging and the Alzheimer's Association sponsored a special task force of prominent researchers in Alzheimer's disease to describe the sequence of events leading to the development of the disease.[2] A lot of the information they used to map this process was based on brain-imaging techniques, such as magnetic resonance imaging (MRI) and positron emission tomography (PET). From these images, we know that the first signs of brain dysfunction occur in the synaptic transmission of neurons. The accumulation of amyloid plaques in the brain also occurs early in the disease process. In fact, there is a great deal of amyloid plaque accumulation before the neurons begin to show evidence of injury through tangled tau proteins. These telltale signs of neuronal injury and death eventually show up on brain imaging as shrinking of the hippocampus and other regions of the brain. Signs of decline in cognitive abilities follow. The rate at which cognitive abilities decline to levels that are characteristic of mild cognitive impairment and dementia varies greatly from person to person.

Vascular Dementia

Vascular dementia is the second most common form of dementia and is a prime example of how diseases and conditions involving the cardiovascular system can bring about disease in the brain. The brain is nourished by a dense network of blood vessels, and about a quarter of the blood that is pumped from the heart is delivered to the brain through this vast arterial system. Blood provides oxygen and fuel to the billions of cells in the brain. Some individuals with dementia have pathologies in the brain that are caused by vascular disease, including obstructions of circulation within the small arteries of the brain or damaged brain tissue caused by strokes. Vascular dementia caused by stroke is more likely to present as an abrupt decrease in cognitive abilities as opposed to the slow, progressive decline that occurs with Alzheimer's dementia. Symptoms of the brain injury can be observed in just a few days and, depending on the region of the brain where the stroke occurred, may result in a sudden loss in the ability to use language appropriately or to name common objects (keys, door, cat) correctly.

PROTECTING AGAINST DEMENTIA THROUGH COGNITIVE RESERVE

When you have a thought, smell a rose, or walk a step, your neurons are involved. They talk to one another through networks of synaptic connections. A synapse is the gap between two neurons in which either an electrical or chemical signal passes from one neuron to the other. There are about one hundred billion neurons in our brains and one hundred to five hundred trillion synapses. Each neuron may have thousands of synaptic connections. Proteins are involved in both the release of the signal (presynaptic protein) and the receipt of that signal (postsynaptic protein). One way that scientists study brain health and function is to analyze brain tissue in the laboratory to quantify the number of these synaptic proteins. These studies have shown that there are fewer synaptic proteins in the brains of people with dementia as well as in people without dementia whose thinking abilities have declined. Nutrients are one of the body's natural defense mechanisms against the loss of synaptic proteins. For example, DHA in the neuronal membrane helps maintain the normal structure and functioning of the neuron, and vitamin E in the neuronal membrane can quickly neutralize free-radical molecules that are generated as the neuron works to transmit signals to other neurons.

One of the more surprising findings in the world of Alzheimer's research is that a large number of people who have significant numbers of plaques and tangles in the brain never progress to clinically manifest the disease. In fact, in studies conducted at the Alzheimer's Disease Center of Rush University, about one-third of individuals who have a diagnosis of Alzheimer's disease, based on the severity of neuropathologies in their brains, have no clinical evidence of the disease. Their cognitive abilities were intact up until their death. These study participants had been tested extensively on an annual basis, completing nineteen cognitive tests and undergoing a neurological examination, and yet they did not show evidence of dementia. It wasn't until *after* their deaths that scientists discovered that their brains were filled with plaques and tangles! A prevailing theory for why this happens is that these individuals have greater neural reserve — that is, an abundance of neurons and synaptic connections that allows the brain to function by *going around* the diseased neurons and brain pathologies. The theory of neural reserve is thought to be the underlying mechanism that explains why participating in cognitive and social activities is associated with lower risk of developing dementia. In other words, activities that stimulate the brain, like doing crossword puzzles, playing bridge, and learning how to play a musical instrument, protect against the cognitive dysfunction associated with dementia by increasing the number of synaptic connections so that the brain can function normally despite the presence of plaques and tangles. Based on what we have learned from animal studies, it is also quite possible that certain nutrients, such as DHA and vitamin E, grow neural reserve by increasing synaptic connections and decreasing neuronal injury and death.

THE ROLE OF OXIDATIVE STRESS AND INFLAMMATION

It's believed that the process of plaque and tangle formation is caused by accumulated damage to neuron cells as a result of oxidative stress and inflammation. Oxidation is a natural phenomenon that occurs when single molecules with a free electron, also known as free radicals, are released in chemical interactions of the brain. Single molecules of oxygen are a common free radical in the brain. Free radical molecules are generated as part of normal metabolic processes, but there are also external sources of free radicals, like smoking, poor diet, infection, and air pollution. The body has natural defense mechanisms to minimize the damage that free radicals have on the brain, and nutrients are fundamental to this process. Vitamin E is one of the more important antioxidant nutrients in the brain. A key to lowering oxidative stress is to consume a diet abundant in antioxidant nutrients and at the same time minimize your body's exposure to free radicals by avoiding fried foods, saturated fats, and smoking.

Inflammation is another natural and healthy process that is designed to defend the body from harmful pathogens or injuries. But too much inflammation is a bad thing. When a tissue is injured, the cells initiate an inflammatory response that attacks the injury's cause, clears the damaged tissue, and gets to work repairing the insult. The problem occurs when damage to the tissue becomes chronic. Thankfully, we now know some of the triggers of chronic inflammation: abdominal fat, obesity, high blood sugar, high LDL blood cholesterol, high triglyceride levels, and high blood pressure. Even better, these are all factors that most of us can control through diet, exercise, and getting enough sleep.

HEALTH AND LIFESTYLE FACTORS LINKED TO BRAIN HEALTH

The factors that have been linked to a decreased risk of dementia are maintaining a healthy diet, managing cardiovascular-related health conditions, exercising, getting quality sleep, participating in activities that are cognitively and socially stimulating, and having a positive response to life stressors and overall outlook on life.

When I say "decreased risk," I do not mean that you will avoid dementia altogether but that your chances of getting the disease will be somewhat lower. An individual may still get Alzheimer's disease even though they lead a pristine life in terms of having an excellent diet; being active physically, socially, and cognitively; and having no chronic diseases or excess weight. This is true for most chronic diseases that have multiple contributing causes, including heart disease, diabetes, and hypertension. We are still learning what all the factors are that increase or decrease one's risk of dementia. There may be predisposing genetic characteristics, risk due to exposure to environmental hazards, or other unknown risk factors that we have yet to learn about. But in general, most people who follow these healthy lifestyle behaviors, and keep chronic conditions under control, will reduce their chances of developing dementia later in life. And for those who might eventually be unfortunate enough to fall victim to the disease for whatever reason, following these healthy lifestyle behaviors will likely result in delayed onset.

Leaving aside diet, which I'll discuss at length in chapter 2, let's explore some of the known risk factors of dementia.

Cardiovascular-Related Health Conditions

One of the most useful and fascinating data findings has been that many of the factors that reduce the risk of developing Alzheimer's disease and cognitive decline are also known to be important for having a robust and healthy heart. In fact, each of the major cardiovascular risk factors that lead to heart disease and stroke — high blood pressure, abnormal blood cholesterol levels, obesity, and diabetes — has also been linked to an increased risk of developing dementia and of increasing decline in cognitive abilities with age. This means that if you work to prevent one disease, you are simultaneously working to ward off the others. There are many effective medications that can control these conditions and reduce your risk of increased cognitive decline or of developing dementia. However, each of these conditions can be largely controlled through diet, exercise, maintaining a healthy weight, and getting quality sleep.

In one rare study that compared a lifestyle intervention with drug therapy for preventing diabetes, the lifestyle intervention won! The study, called the Diabetes Prevention Program, randomly assigned 3,234 obese prediabetics to treatment with metformin, a diabetes medication, or to a program of diet and exercise designed to decrease body weight by 7 percent.[3] At the end of three years, the incidence of diabetes was reduced by 58 percent with the lifestyle intervention and by 31 percent with metformin, as compared with a placebo.

Obesity in middle age has been linked to greater cognitive decline and to increased risk of dementia in later years. Therefore, it is important to control weight early in life, even though it gets harder and harder as we age. A natural process of growing older is loss in lean body mass, including muscles, organs, and bones, and an increase in fat tissue. With the loss in lean tissue comes a decrease in water. Joints and arteries stiffen. The greater accumulation of fat occurs in the mid-region, especially around the internal organs. (Think of the middle-aged "beer gut.") This process begins around the age of thirty. From age forty to seventy, the average loss in height is about a half inch every ten years, with greater reductions after age seventy. An average person can expect to lose up to three inches in height by old age and amass one-third more fat tissue compared with young adulthood. Although it is by no means inevitable, most people gain weight up to the age of fifty-five for men and sixty-five for women. Then the process of weight loss begins, due largely to the fact that fat weighs less than muscle. The extent of these later life changes in fat and lean tissue depends on diet and physical activity, lifestyle behaviors that are in our control, so watching our diet and making a routine of aerobic and strength exercises will minimize the amount of weight gain and loss in lean mass that comes with aging.

A number of studies conducted in industrialized countries like the United States have shown that changes in blood cholesterol and blood pressure mirror the weight increases from young to old adulthood. Blood cholesterol begins to rise around age twenty until about age sixty or sixty-five. Total cholesterol levels tend to be higher for men than for women before age fifty, but after age fifty, when women transition into menopause, the levels are higher for women. Cardiovascular risk increases when LDL cholesterol, the bad cholesterol that builds up in the arteries, is greater than 130 mg/dL, and when HDL cholesterol, the good cholesterol that helps remove the bad cholesterol from the arteries, is less than 50 mg/dL. According to the Centers for Disease Control and Prevention, 31.7 percent of the US adult population has high LDL cholesterol, and only one in every three of these adults has their cholesterol under control.

Blood pressure follows a similar aging pattern. Before age fifty-five, men have a higher prevalence of hypertension, but after menopause, women exceed men in prevalence of the disease. As we age, our arteries tend to become less elastic, so that the heart has to work harder to pump blood; this causes a rise in the pressure of the blood through the arteries. For this reason, systolic hypertension (the higher number) is more common than diastolic hypertension in old age. The Joint National Committee on the Prevention, Detection, Evaluation, and Treatment of Blood Pressure defined hypertension as blood pressure levels greater than 140/90 mmHg. A whopping 80 percent of the US population sixty-five and older has blood pressure levels in the hypertension range.

During a time when one drug trial after another has failed to show effectiveness for the treatment of cognitive impairment and Alzheimer's disease, the dementia field was stunned by a 2015 report of a Finnish trial demonstrating reductions in cognitive decline through management of vascular risk factors and lifestyle interventions. The trial, called FINGER (Finnish Geriatric Intervention Study to Prevent Cognitive Impairment and Disability) randomly assigned 1,260 older individuals age sixty to ninety to one of two groups.[4] One group received counseling to improve their diet, increase their exercise levels, participate in cognitive training, and monitor their blood pressure and weight. The control group received advice on the importance of these lifestyle and health factors in maintaining cognitive abilities but did not receive the intensive attention to individual lifestyle changes or the opportunities to participate in exercise and cognitive training programs. After two years, the group that received the multipronged program to improve lifestyle behaviors and address vascular risk had significantly less decline in cognitive test scores compared with the simple advice group.

Another fascinating study compared the risk factors for dementia in an African American population living in Indianapolis, Indiana, and a Yoruba population living in Ibadan, Nigeria.[5] They found that weight and levels of blood pressure and blood cholesterol were much lower in the Nigerian population than in the Indianapolis one. The prevalence of diabetes was also lower. The low rates of cardiovascular conditions were likely influenced by the mostly vegetarian diet of the Nigerian population. The low-calorie, low-fat diet consisted primarily of tubers or roots like yams and cassava, grains such as rice, and small amounts of fish. Fish is the major source of protein in the Nigerian diet, primarily herring, tilapia, mackerel, and catfish. The body mass index (BMI) among the Nigerians was on average 22 in females and 21 in males. This compared to BMIs of 29.8 and 28.3 for females and males, respectively, in the Indianapolis African American population. A particularly striking finding in this study was that the rate of dementia in the African Americans was nearly *three times higher* than that in the Yoruba! This is an amazing contrast when you consider the advanced medical and environmental technologies and treatments that we have in the United States that aren't available in Nigeria.

Finally, in long-term studies of dementia that followed individuals all the way from middle to late adult years, those who developed dementia later in life had the highest levels of blood pressure, blood cholesterol, and obesity during middle age. And what is particularly interesting is that for each of these vascular conditions, there was a much steeper decline in the levels in the late adult years among those who contracted dementia, so that after age seventy-five the levels were actually lower than in the individuals who remained dementia-free. We don't fully understand why this might occur, but these factors are interrelated, and one of the consequences of dementia is weight loss.

Obesity, blood pressure, and blood cholesterol level are greatly affected by diet. Taking strategic and nutritious steps, then, will have an undeniable impact on how fast you age and on your health over the long term. You can't argue with the numbers, and science tells us over and over that diet and exercise will help you significantly decrease the age-related increases in blood cholesterol, blood pressure, and weight—and decrease age-related declines in brain function. When you give your body what it needs to thrive, you can't help but benefit in the immediate and long term.

Exercise

It is remarkable how diet and physical activity are at the root of nearly all major chronic conditions and diseases. Focusing on these two basic components of daily living is key to aging healthfully. Physical activity and aerobic fitness are critical to maintaining a healthy cardiovascular system as well as a healthy brain. Aerobic fitness results in less shrinkage of the brain with age and slower decline in cognitive abilities.

It is not possible yet to target a minimum number of hours or number of times per week of physical activity for maintaining brain health. What we do know is that aerobic activity and aerobic fitness are better than nonaerobic forms of exercise, such as weight lifting. Aerobic activities like walking, running, swimming, and cycling use your large muscles in a rhythmic way for a sustained period of time, which requires the heart to pump blood to deliver oxygen to your working muscles. These activities improve the performance of your heart and lungs, especially if your activity is intense enough to increase your heart rate to the point that you're out of breath. Nonaerobic activities simply aren't as effective because they typically don't last as long and don't require the heart to fuel the muscles with oxygen. Whereas nonaerobic exercise has been demonstrated to benefit older adults by strengthening muscles and bones and improving coordination, thereby reducing the occurrence of falls and improving mobility, it is the improvement of circulation to the brain that aerobic activity affords as well as the ramped-up production of certain hormones (such as BDNF, or brain-derived neurotrophic factor) that protect cognition and stimulate neuron growth.

In one clinical trial, 120 older adults without dementia were randomly assigned to moderate-intensity aerobic exercise or to stretching and toning three days per week.[6] MRIs of the brain were conducted at the beginning of the trial and again after six months and one year. After a year, the stretching control group experienced a 1.4 percent decrease in the volume of the hippocampus, the region of the brain associated with memory, but the aerobic exercise group had a 2 percent increase in hippocampal volume. Greater increases in hippocampal volume were correlated with both improvements in aerobic fitness level over the one-year interval and with increases in BDNF. Further, increased hippocampal volume was directly related to improvements in memory performance. In other words, taking brisk walks on a regular basis may help you avoid those annoying memory lapses when you are unable to retrieve words in a conversation or remember names at a social function.

Sleep

Sleep is another lifestyle factor that has been found to impact the brain. Numerous studies have shown that loss of sleep impairs memory, attention, and the ability to problem solve at any age. Furthermore, fragmented and poor-quality sleep in our older years has been associated with faster cognitive decline and greater risks of Alzheimer's disease and stroke. The recommendation that adults get seven to eight hours of sleep a night to maintain good physical and cognitive health is linked to studies that observed lower rates of a number of chronic diseases — including heart disease, diabetes, stroke, and cognitive impairment — with adequate sleep. So, it makes good sense to do your best to meet this requirement.

As we age, our sleep patterns change, even though the total time required for sleep does not change. Our sleep is more easily interrupted, we get up more frequently during the night, and the period of deep sleep decreases. Our internal clocks change so that we tend to get sleepy earlier in the evening and to wake earlier in the morning. In addition to these changes, the aging process causes the tissues lining our airways to sag, just as our skin begins to sag, and this increases the tendency to snore and the development of sleep apnea, conditions that can decrease the amount of oxygen that gets to the brain. Severe apnea has been shown to have harmful effects on brain tissue, leading to neuronal cell death and impaired function. Sleep apnea is very common with older age, affecting as many as two-thirds of adults age sixty-five and older, and excess weight is the strongest predictor.

Research on sleep and the brain is relatively new, but some exciting new discoveries suggest that it is during sleep that toxins, like the abnormal proteins that form Alzheimer's plaques, are flushed from the brain.

How do we make sure that we get the restorative benefits of sleep? Sleep experts recommend instituting a regular routine of to-bed and to-wake times, getting daily exercise and outdoor light exposure during the day, and restricting coffee consumption to before noon and alcohol to no later than two to three hours before bedtime. Sleep medications may work, but experts warn that regular use can actually impair the ability to sleep soundly and can even diminish cognitive functioning.

There's no question that it is important to put more effort into maintaining good lifestyle habits as you age, because it becomes more and more challenging to get good quality sleep, maintain a healthy weight, and keep your body running efficiently.

Cognitive and Social Activities

There have been a lot of studies on cognitive activities and exercises to maintain cognitive abilities with age. Most have found that participation in any intellectual activity—for example, reading books and newspapers, doing crossword puzzles, playing games or musical instruments—slows decline in cognitive abilities. Several randomized trials have tested the effectiveness of various cognitive exercises in preventing decline in abilities. The results of these trials have indicated that the exercises were effective but that they were very specific and did not translate into other areas of cognitive functioning. For example, cognitive training in memory does not appear to improve the ability to solve problems. For well-rounded enrichment, you need to mix up your activities. Learning a new skill that is both fun and challenging can be particularly effective; try learning a new language or learning how to play a new musical instrument. Challenging the brain with cognitive activities is key.

Keeping socially active and having a purpose in life have also been found to protect against cognitive decline with age and the development of dementia. Brain-healthy social activities involve interacting with others in ways that make you feel connected, participating in purposeful activities with others, and maintaining meaningful social relationships. In our Chicago studies, the participants who were frequently socially active had 70 percent less decline in their cognitive abilities compared to those who were infrequently active.[7] However, if the interactions with others were negative, greater cognitive impairment and faster decline resulted.[8] In addition, the participants who expressed loneliness had a faster rate of cognitive decline, and the risk of Alzheimer's disease was more than doubled.[9] What this means for you and your mind is that any increased stimulation that occurs in a social setting should be positive. Attending dinners with family — one of my favorite pastimes — is a great example of an activity that maintains brain function (unless, of course, the interactions with family are stressful or negative).

Positive Outlook on Life

Personality characteristics can also affect the brain. Having a positive response to life stressors and overall outlook on life has been related to lower risk of dementia. In our Rush studies, those participants who were more prone to psychological distress (they had a tendency to be tense and jittery, and worriers) declined at a faster rate than those who experienced low distress.[10] By contrast, the participants who expressed a greater sense of purpose in life and felt good about their lives and their future were significantly less likely to develop Alzheimer's disease.[11]

After reading this chapter, you should be getting the idea that you have a lot of control over how well you age. Leading an active life — cognitively, physically, and socially — can lower your chance of developing dementia, as can maintaining healthy levels of weight, blood pressure, blood cholesterol, and sleep. The remaining chapters of the book provide an understanding of how diet plays a key role in all these factors, and what basic steps you need to follow to keep your brain healthy.

CHAPTER 2

Essential Nutrients for the Brain

Your brain is an incredibly voracious organ—an area of high metabolic activity and a high turnover of nutrients. And even though it is just one of many organs in your body, it uses 20 percent of the calories you consume at rest to carry out its daily functions! Roughly a third of that energy is used to rejuvenate the brain and clear away damaged proteins and cells. Every thought you have, movement you make, and sense you use (hearing, sight, sound, smell, and touch) requires the neurons in your brain to work—and this demands a lot of fuel and nutrients. Thus, the brain has a great need for nutrients that help it survive and thrive.

There are two basic categories of nutrients: macronutrients, which provide the structural components as well as the fuel required for cells to function, and micronutrients, which are needed to build and repair tissues and to protect the cells from damage caused as the brain uses energy to function. In order for your brain to function at its best, you have to keep replenishing your nutrients.

The brain regulates which nutrients and how much of those nutrients it will allow in and out of this vital organ. It does this primarily through the blood-brain barrier—a semipermeable membrane that separates the brain's circulating blood from the extracellular fluid in the central nervous system. In a sense, the blood-brain barrier acts as a gatekeeper to the brain, selectively letting some nutrients in and blocking other harmful substances from entering (certain sugars like sucrose, for instance, are not allowed to cross the barrier).

Some nutrients have special transport systems that usher them directly into the brain. For example, the alpha tocopherol form of vitamin E has its own transport protein that latches onto only this specific vitamin E form and delivers it directly to the brain and other organs. For reasons that scientists do not understand, there are no special proteins for other forms of vitamin E, even though they get into the brain and have important roles to play. DHA is also essential to the structure and functioning of the brain and easily penetrates the blood-brain barrier. And then there are trace elements like copper, zinc, and iron that are essential for normal brain function and development, but an imbalance of these elements can be harmful. Excess levels of these biometals play a central role in Alzheimer's disease through the formation and neurotoxicity of beta amyloid and neurofibrillary tangles. There is much to discover about the blood-brain barrier and its role in nutrition and the aging brain. Suffice it to say that as we age, every organ system of the body is aging, and that includes the blood-brain barrier. But there are many things we can do to keep this gatekeeper running efficiently, including maintaining a healthy diet and exercising regularly.

In this chapter, I will describe the most important nutrients required to keep the brain functioning at its peak based on the best scientific evidence to date. These nutrients are all featured in Laura's mind-enriching and delicious recipes in part II of the book. In addition to the established brain-healthy nutrients, I will also discuss the foods and dietary components that either have moderate or limited scientific evidence for brain health or that have no evidence but are touted for their positive effects on brain health. Included among the latter group are vitamin D, coconut oil, resveratrol, and ginkgo biloba. It is important that you understand which of the latest fads are backed up by scientific evidence, because there is a lot of "junk science" out there in the media. I know, because I speak frequently to the public about nutrition and the brain, and I am always asked about the latest nutrient or superfood to cure Alzheimer's disease. I've tried to cover all of these in this chapter. Of course, vitamin supplements come up a lot. I give special attention to this topic at the end of the chapter.

FILL YOUR PLATE WITH ANTIOXIDANTS, B VITAMINS, AND HEALTHY FATS

Why Antioxidant Nutrients Matter So Much

As we saw in chapter 1, oxidative damage is known to be involved in what goes wrong in the brain to cause neurodegenerative diseases like Alzheimer's disease. But if we broaden the perspective, free radicals involved in this damage are said to play an even greater role in how we age. In fact, the Free Radical Theory of Aging states that accumulated damage to cells from free radical molecules gradually breaks down the body systems, including those related to the brain.

So why are free radicals so dangerous? In most molecules, the electrons, which are negatively charged, are paired and balanced by the positively charged protons in the molecule's nucleus. A free radical molecule, however, has an unpaired electron, and this makes the molecule very unstable. Like a live wire, it's highly reactive and can damage cells. The chemical processes that use oxygen tend to create free radical molecules that can injure brain cells. Because your brain is a site of high metabolic activity and uses a lot of oxygen to function, it is particularly vulnerable to oxidative damage.

While free radicals are generated as part of normal bodily functions—for example, when you digest food, breathe, grow, and fight infection—they're also caused by environmental insults, such as contact with pollutants, smoking, and viruses. Free radicals can also run amok when you contract an illness like cancer, heart disease, diabetes, or obesity. Thankfully, your body has natural defense mechanisms to combat free radicals, called antioxidant enzymes and antioxidant nutrients. Even the antioxidant enzymes are composed of various nutrients. You can see, then, how imperative nutrients are to fighting age-inducing free radicals and preserving your body through the years—and why it's crucial to replenish them as best you can.

What's more, despite the high metabolic activity of the brain, this organ has relatively few antioxidant enzymes and nutrients compared to other body organs. Vitamin E is one of the primary antioxidant nutrients in the brain and lives within the neuron cell's membrane. It's there to snap up free radical molecules as they're generated and prevent damage to the cells that could disrupt their functioning. Numerous studies in animals and humans demonstrate the important role of vitamin E in the brain as an antioxidant and anti-inflammatory that protects against oxidative damage to neurons and the development of the amyloid plaques that define Alzheimer's disease. These studies have also found that vitamin E preserves memory and other cognitive abilities and reduces the risk of developing Alzheimer's disease. Most of the studies have focused on just the alpha tocopherol form of vitamin E, the richest sources of which are nuts, seeds, and oils. This form of vitamin E is also traditionally the only form found in vitamin supplements. Of the other tocopherol forms—beta, delta, and gamma—gamma tocopherol has also been found to have anti-inflammatory and antioxidant properties. It is the main tocopherol consumed in the US diet, largely thanks to the high amount in soybean and corn oils, which are often used in packaged foods.

Other antioxidant nutrients include carotenoids, flavonoids and other polyphenols, and vitamin C, though their roles in human brain function are less well understood. Vitamin C is an antioxidant nutrient that circulates within the plasma but also helps restore vitamin E to its antioxidant capacity. Some of the richest food sources of vitamin C include citrus fruits, tomatoes, potatoes, sweet peppers, strawberries, and cantaloupes. Of the carotenoids, beta-carotene and lutein have been specifically linked to dementia prevention. These carotenoids are abundant in leafy green vegetables and in orange and yellow vegetables. A wide range of foods and beverages — chocolate, spices, fruits, vegetables, tea, coffee, wine — contain the very large group of flavonoids and other polyphenols.

Whereas there is little scientific evidence to support vitamin C as being protective of the brain, beta-carotene and lutein are highly promising. Levels of these two carotenoid nutrients have been measured in the human brain and are particularly abundant in the brain region that is involved in eye function. The findings from epidemiological studies that have examined cognition and dietary beta-carotene are not consistent, and it is not clear why some studies show positive benefits while others show no association. One very large randomized trial, however, demonstrated that 50 milligrams of a beta-carotene vitamin supplement taken every other day for eighteen years resulted in better performance on cognitive tests among 4,052 participants of the Physicians' Health Study II.[12] There was no effect among the 1,904 trial participants who took the beta-carotene supplement for only one year, which suggests that long-term exposure to beta-carotene is required for brain health.

Although the studies that have examined lutein are limited, there is good scientific evidence that links this dietary component to better cognitive functioning and decreased risk of dementia. One such study conducted in the Bordeaux region of France measured blood levels of carotenoids in 1,092 community residents without dementia and followed them over ten years to see who developed dementia.[13] Of all the various types of carotenoids, only lutein was associated with a reduced risk of developing Alzheimer's dementia by 24 percent. And in my diet study of 960 older Chicago residents, we observed that those participants who had the highest dietary intake of lutein from food sources had significantly slower decline in their cognitive abilities. Kale, spinach, and collards are three great sources of lutein.

Flavonoids represent one class of polyphenols that can be further categorized into a number of subclasses, including flavanones (good sources: citrus fruits), flavones (artichokes, green bell peppers), flavonols (radishes, cranberries, onions), anthocyanins (blueberries, red wine, red cabbage), and flavanols (cocoa, dark chocolate, black tea, green tea). Only a few epidemiological studies have investigated dietary intakes of flavonoids, and they have consistently shown positive benefits for reducing cognitive decline and Alzheimer's disease. Studies from animal models indicate that flavonoids may be responsible for reducing neuroinflammation in the brain. This is a relatively new area of research because data on the levels of flavonoids in various foods have only recently become available.

Fuel Up on B Vitamins

As I mentioned earlier in the book, vitamin B_{12} plays a crucial role in the brain's normal functioning. One of the symptoms of vitamin B_{12} deficiency syndrome, in fact, is memory impairment. Vitamin B_{12} is also a co-factor with two other B vitamins, folate (vitamin B_9) and vitamin B_6, in the metabolism of the amino acid homocysteine. Deficiencies in either folate or vitamin B_{12} increase homocysteine levels, and high levels of homocysteine in the blood can cause inflammation and atherosclerosis. Atherosclerosis, the buildup of fats, cholesterol, and other substances in artery walls, has been linked to an increased risk of coronary heart disease, stroke, and dementia. Although a direct tie to the brain or its neuropathologies has not been established for folate or vitamin B_6, study after study has shown that those with low dietary intake or blood levels of folate are associated with increased risk of developing Alzheimer's disease.

So how can you get your fill of these essential nutrients? The richest food sources of folate are yeast, beans, poultry, cereals and whole grains, nuts and seeds, and leafy green vegetables. Vitamin B_6 is found in many foods but is highest in seafood, poultry, beans, egg yolks, beef, and fortified cereals. An individual's nutrient status in folate and vitamin B_6 can be readily addressed by eating more of these foods, but be careful not to take in too much folic acid, the supplement form of folate, as a means of compensating. A number of studies, including my own Chicago studies, have found that taking folic acid supplements may actually *increase* cognitive decline in people whose vitamin B_{12} levels are inadequate. And while I think it's better to take in your vitamins through food, it's much harder to do this with vitamin B_{12}, especially as you age. Older age, medication use, alcohol consumption, and a condition known as pernicious anemia can significantly impair how well you absorb vitamin B_{12} from food sources. Thus, attempts to improve vitamin B_{12} nutrient levels through diet are less likely to be successful, and middle-aged and older adults should have their levels checked by their doctor. If they are low, the doctor may recommend vitamin supplements or monthly injections to help restore vitamin B_{12} to optimum levels.

Focus on the Right Dietary Fats

There are three basic types of fat in the human diet: saturated, monounsaturated, and polyunsaturated. Polyunsaturated fats can be further categorized into omega-6 and omega-3 fatty acids. A major distinction among these fats is that saturated fat is solid at room temperature, whereas mono- and polyunsaturated fats are liquid at room temperature. A diet that is substantially higher in mono- and polyunsaturated fats than saturated fats results in a favorable blood cholesterol profile that is high in the good cholesterol (HDL) and low in the bad cholesterol (LDL). This type of dietary fat composition is known to reduce atherosclerosis and the risk of heart disease and stroke. Although the science is much less developed on the effects of fat composition on dementia, it appears that the same is likely true here, too.

In 2014, one seriously flawed study concluded that saturated fat was not responsible for increased risk of heart disease, which threw everyone in the nutrition and medical community into a justified tizzy. The study received a great deal of attention in the media but was strongly refuted by the most reputable scientists in the field. The argument for limiting saturated fat intake is backed up by consistent and high-quality scientific evidence. Rest assured that the scientific literature is clear in its conclusion that diets that are higher in saturated fat and lower in the unsaturated fats *increase* cardiovascular diseases and risk of death. A very important distinction to make here is that calories from saturated fat intake need to be replaced by healthier fats, which we'll discuss in a bit, and not by increasing caloric intake from sugars. An unfortunate consequence of the food industry's response to a demand for lower saturated fats in food products is that they increased the sugar content substantially. The craze in recent years for food products labeled "no fat" or "low fat" has greatly increased consumption of sugar in the United States. Sugar has little nutritious value, but there is limited scientific evidence that it is bad for the brain.

But let's get back to fats. In my Chicago study, I found that individuals who consumed the highest amount of saturated fat in their diets had *double* the risk of developing Alzheimer's disease.[14] They also experienced the fastest decline in their cognitive abilities over six years, compared with those in the study who had the lowest consumption of saturated fat.[15] In this study, there was also evidence that high consumption of polyunsaturated and monounsaturated fats was associated with a lower risk of Alzheimer's disease and slower decline in cognitive abilities. Not surprisingly, the highest sources of saturated fat in the US diet are pizza and cheese, as well as other high-fat dairy products and red meats. And while grass-fed meats are, in some circles, considered to be a kind of loophole for healthy red meat consumption, in our current state of research, there is no evidence to support the idea that grass-fed meats are any different from grain-fed when it comes to red meat's impact on brain health. The studies to examine this have not yet been done.

As for healthy sources of unsaturated fats, look to vegetable oils, nuts/seeds, and fish to give you the most bang for your buck. These foods also contain some saturated fat, but you definitely shouldn't avoid them for that reason. I am often asked about whether the brain benefits from oils that are higher in polyunsaturated fats (such as safflower or canola oil) or monounsaturated fats (such as olive oil). The answer is not clear at this point in the research on dementia. Keep in mind, though, that extra-virgin olive oil, a rich source of monounsaturated fats, does have the additional benefit of polyphenols, which have antioxidant and anti-inflammatory properties. Olive oil has also been shown to increase HDL (good) cholesterol. In PREDIMED (Prevención con Dieta Mediterránea), a landmark study conducted in Spain, participants were randomly assigned to the Mediterranean diet or to a low-fat diet to assess the effects of the Mediterranean diet on the prevention of cardiovascular disease.[16] (We'll explore the Mediterranean diet in more detail in chapter 6.) Some of the participants were asked to consume three to four tablespoons daily of extra-virgin olive oil. Sure enough, these subjects performed significantly better on cognitive tests compared with the group on the low-fat diet. Using extra-virgin olive oil, then, as the primary oil in your home may help improve your heart and brain health. I use it to sauté my vegetables, and at restaurants I ask for olive oil to put on my bread instead of butter.

Omega-3 fatty acids are vital to the brain and normal brain function. They are found primarily in nuts, seeds, oils, and seafood. Alpha-linolenic acid, one of the omega-3s, is considered to be an "essential nutrient" — that is, a nutrient that is necessary for human function but must be consumed because it cannot be produced within the human body. Alpha-linolenic acid is found in walnuts, flaxseed, rapeseed, soybeans, chia seeds, and the oils from these nuts and seeds. A considerable amount of research on the omega-3 fatty acids has shown them to be instrumental in neurocognitive development beginning in utero and continuing through the early childhood years. This research was first initiated by the observation that human milk is abundant in omega-3 fatty acids. Scientists wanted to understand what role these fatty acids play in human health, especially because the first infant formulas did not contain them. This research established a sound physiological basis for the saying that "fish is brain food." The primary structure of the brain is lipid material (a type of fat), and the primary brain lipid is DHA—a long-chain omega-3 fatty acid that can be directly consumed from seafood sources or metabolized from alpha-linolenic acid. DHA is particularly abundant in the most metabolically active areas of the brain: the cerebral cortex, the synaptic terminals, and the mitochondria, an organelle of the neuron cell that supplies its energy. As we age, DHA levels in the brain decrease due to oxidative stress. In studies of aged rodents, diets rich in DHA resulted in increased brain levels. However, in humans the conversion rate from alpha-linolenic acid to DHA is very low (less than 1 percent), so it's controversial whether you can obtain the same levels of DHA through non-seafood sources.

THE JURY'S OUT ON CURCUMIN, GINKGO BILOBA, RESVERATROL, AND VITAMIN D

Curcumin: Promising but Unproven

Curcumin is a polyphenolic compound found in turmeric, an East Indian spice that comes from a shrub grown in India, other parts of Asia, and Africa. You are likely familiar with its golden color and warm, bitter taste as one of the identifying characteristics of curry powder and mustard. Turmeric has long been used in Ayurvedic and Chinese medicine to aid digestion and liver function, relieve arthritis pain, and regulate menstruation. It's also traditionally been used as a topical treatment for eczema and wound healing. In recent years, integrative medical communities have lauded it as a treatment for gastrointestinal conditions, dementia, and cancer. Curcumin's potent anti-inflammatory and antioxidant properties have propelled it into the world of westernized medicine, where it's being examined for its potential effects on cancer, inflammatory conditions, and neurodegenerative diseases.

Because of the difficulties of investigating the health benefits of spices through epidemiological studies, research on curcumin has been confined to animal models and randomized trials of pharmacologic preparations. The animal research has shown promise for Alzheimer's and Parkinson's diseases, as rodents administered curcumin have demonstrated better memory function and reduced levels of amyloid plaques, inflammation, oxidative stress, and neuron loss. However, clinical trials of pharmacologic preparations of curcumin in humans have faced challenges due to curcumin's low bioavailability, or the amount that is actually absorbed and reaches the tissues. There are numerous clinical trials in progress with various preparations of drugs containing curcumin. So far, the trials have had limited success, and the scientific evidence falls short to support curcumin as a preventive agent against neurodegenerative and other diseases.

Ginkgo Biloba: Better to Treat Disease Than Prevent It?

Ginkgo biloba, one of the top-selling herbal supplements in the United States, has been repeatedly said to help prevent Alzheimer's disease. It comes from a tree native to China where, historically, the seeds and leaves have been used as food and in traditional medicine. Extracts of ginkgo biloba leaves are high in antioxidant nutritional components such as flavonoids and other polyphenolic compounds, and laboratory studies have shown that ginkgo biloba improves blood flow by opening up blood vessels and reducing the tendency for blood cells to coagulate. It's said to help with blood flow to the legs and, specifically, with Raynaud's syndrome, characterized by the narrowing of blood vessels to the fingers and toes.

Ginkgo biloba has also been used to treat depression, anxiety, head-aches, and tinnitus (ringing in the ears).

That being said, there is strong evidence *against* ginkgo biloba in the prevention of Alzheimer's disease. Two large randomized trials involving nearly six thousand older community residents, one conducted in France[17] and the other in centers across the United States,[18] found no benefit of five to six years of treatment with ginkgo biloba in the prevention of Alzheimer's disease. The US trial also found no evidence that six years of ginkgo biloba treatment prevented cognitive decline or the occurrence of stroke.[19]

However, among patients who already had Alzheimer's disease or vascular dementia, data from randomized trials on ginkgo biloba's therapeutic effects have shown some positive results, although the findings are by no means consistent. More recent trials that are larger and more scientifically sound have not found protective benefits. Because of the inconsistencies, the question remains as to whether and for whom ginkgo biloba may improve cognitive and behavioral symptoms associated with dementia. An important note is that the ginkgo biloba extracts appear to be safe; no trial reported adverse effects.

Resveratrol

Resveratrol has been billed as a surefire protectant against aging and chronic diseases, including Alzheimer's disease, diabetes, and cancer—but let's consider what we know from the science. Resveratrol is a polyphenol contained in the skin of grapes and berries, and in peanuts. You'll also find it in wine—red wine, in particular, since the grapes' skins are part of the winemaking process. Wine's resveratrol content depends on the type of grape used, as well as the region in which it's grown; grapes from France's Bordeaux region, for instance, have the highest concentrations of resveratrol.

In the 1980s, this region was where the medical community's interest in resveratrol began, since residents of the area had a low rate of heart disease despite diets high in saturated fat. This seeming contradiction led researchers to coin the term "French paradox" and to hypothesize that moderate wine consumption lowered the risk of heart disease.

Studies show that moderate wine intake also lowers the risk of developing dementia and slows cognitive decline. However, it's unlikely that resveratrol is the factor in wine responsible for these promising outcomes, because even though the animal studies have found protective effects on the brain, the daily dose used in these studies would be the equivalent of drinking one hundred to one thousand bottles of wine — surely a fatal exercise! Even so, laboratory and animal studies have demonstrated that resveratrol is a potent antioxidant and anti-inflammatory compound that protects against cell death and cancerous cells, which makes it worth mentioning. To date, human studies have been few in number and of short duration, and most were designed to test whether manufactured resveratrol supplements are safe and tolerable. However, there have been no studies to examine whether resveratrol is effective in humans for preventing cognitive decline and chronic disease. Suffice it to say that at this point, resveratrol is an interesting potential neuroprotectant compound, but current evidence doesn't support the idea that it will keep your brain functioning at its peak. This may change as more of the trials in progress report their findings and the science develops.

Vitamin D: Not (Yet) a Magic Bullet for Dementia

Over the past ten years, vitamin D deficiency has been linked to one health condition after another, including osteoporosis, different cancers, diabetes, hypertension, multiple sclerosis, and yes, dementia and Alzheimer's disease. And since it's estimated that about two-thirds of the US population have at best marginal levels of vitamin D, this only heightens the importance of research. In recent years, physicians have begun screening patients for vitamin D insufficiency, and there has been widespread prescribing of D supplements. The thinking goes that at best, it's a magic bullet; at worst, it's a fail-safe precaution.

Yet as more and more studies investigate the health benefits of vitamin D, the weight of scientific evidence simply has not panned out for most conditions except for those related to the bones, such as osteoporosis, fractures, and falls, since the body needs vitamin D for bone growth and bone remodeling. Vitamin D promotes calcium absorption in the gut and, together with calcium, prevents osteoporosis in older adults and rickets in children. In the case of dementia and cognitive decline, it's only been in the last few years that findings from prospective studies have been reported, and the evidence is much too inconsistent to conclude that lack of sufficient vitamin D contributes to neurodegenerative diseases. Neither is there evidence for a strong biological basis between the two. Still, there are multiple, ongoing randomized trials on the effects of vitamin D supplementation on cognitive decline and other conditions of aging that should contribute greatly to our understanding of this important nutrient.

All that said, it may be a good idea to take vitamin D to support bone health, especially if you're at high risk for bone loss; and should the cognitive decline research change, you'll be a step ahead of the game. The current recommended dietary allowance (RDA) is 600 IU per day for adults up to age seventy and 800 IU for those older than seventy. Vitamin D is found in only a few foods: the skin and oil of oily fish like salmon, beef liver, egg yolks, cheese, some mushrooms, and fortified foods like yogurt, cereal, milk, and orange juice. Sun exposure is another great way to get vitamin D. Ultraviolet sun rays are absorbed through the skin and converted to vitamin D. Some vitamin D experts recommend twice-weekly sun exposure of five to thirty minutes between 10:00 a.m. and 3:00 p.m. to absorb sufficient vitamin D for synthesis.

Be aware that there are scenarios in which vitamin D is tough to metabolize. Older individuals and those with dark skin have a harder time doing this through skin exposure. If you have impaired liver and kidney function, you're also more likely to have insufficient levels. Another risk factor for vitamin D insufficiency is obesity, since vitamin D is a fat-soluble vitamin that's stored in fat tissue. People who are obese may have higher dietary requirements because less of the vitamin is circulating and available for other tissues.

ARE VITAMINS FROM SUPPLEMENTS JUST AS EFFECTIVE AS FOOD?

A number of randomized trials have tested the effects on cognitive decline of individual vitamin supplements, including B vitamins, vitamins E and C, fish oil, and multivitamins. Most of the vitamin supplement trials have not found positive effects on cognition, but most of them also have a consistent flaw in the trial design that makes it tricky to believe the findings.

First, in US vitamin supplement trials, it's common practice for scientists to ignore the participants' existing nutrient status going into the trials. It's also common to allow all the subjects to take a multivitamin during the trial, whether or not they are randomly assigned to the vitamin supplement treatment group. This has the effect of raising the nutrient status of all the study participants to adequate levels. As a result, the US trials to date have tested only whether *therapeutically* high doses of vitamins are beneficial in comparison to nutritionally adequate levels. And those dose levels may be sixty to ninety times the recommended dietary levels you'd obtain through foods.

Such questionable design ignores a basic principal of nutrition science, which is that the human body functions optimally at some intermediate level of a nutrient. Nutrient levels that fall below or above this level can result in marginal physiological functioning or even death, depending on the nutrient. This is perhaps why the vitamin trials have yielded negative findings — they haven't been designed to correct or raise insufficient or marginal vitamin status to the optimum normal range.

To conduct a valid test of whether a nutrient is important in a disease process, the clinical trials should be designed to include only those individuals who have *insufficient levels* of the nutrient and then to supplement them with the nutrient of interest. If there is indeed a relationship between the nutrient and the disease or health outcome, the contrast in the nutrient levels between the treated and control groups will be more likely to show a significant effect. Without question, you'll be able to see whether the supplemented individuals are raised from sub-optimum to optimum levels of physiological functioning.

By way of example, let's consider whether vitamin E has an effect on dementia. Numerous laboratory and animal studies have demonstrated the antioxidant and anti-inflammatory effects of vitamin E on neurons and its promotion of healthy brain function and protection against Alzheimer's disease neuropathology. This forms a strong biological basis for the role of vitamin E in dementia prevention. Many epidemiological studies in different populations around the world have observed associations of vitamin E in diet and biochemical measures of blood with preserved cognition and lower risk of Alzheimer's disease.

Now let's consider the evidence on vitamin E from randomized clinical trials, which you would also expect to show preventive effects if there is a true benefit of vitamin E on the brain. To date, a number of randomized trials of vitamin E effects on dementia have been conducted in the United States, and the results have been inconsistent. Two of the trials were conducted in patients who already had Alzheimer's disease,[20, 21] one trial was of patients with mild cognitive impairment,[22] and two others were prevention trials conducted in people who had no evidence of cognitive impairment.[23, 24] A very high dose of 2,000 IU of vitamin E was used in the trials of Alzheimer's disease. No effect was observed on cognitive decline (such as memory), but in both studies positive benefits on functional decline (like getting dressed) were observed. The vitamin E supplement was effective in reducing the rate of decline in activities of daily living, hours that a caregiver needed to be present, and whether subjects were admitted into nursing homes. This high therapeutic dose of vitamin E was also used in the study of participants with mild cognitive impairment, but there was no effect of the vitamin E supplementation on the progression to Alzheimer's disease or on cognitive decline. It is important to distinguish these trials as therapeutic interventions to combat the disease; the nutrient supplement was a pharmacologic dose of vitamin E that is ninety times the recommended dietary levels.

A much different relationship exists between nutrients and normal physiological functioning in the absence of disease. The two trials that investigated the effect of vitamin E supplements on cognitive change in individuals without evidence of dementia used dose levels of 600 IU every other day.[23, 24] Neither trial found an effect of vitamin E on cognitive decline in the subjects overall. Yet in one of the trials, there was a statistically significant protective benefit from the high-dose vitamin E in those participants whose dietary intake of vitamin E was very low (less than 9 IU per day, or less than half the RDA of 22 IU per day).[24]

Does the fact that the prevention trials found no effect on cognitive decline or progression to Alzheimer's disease mean that the animal and epidemiological studies are wrong and that the epidemiological studies are all biased? I don't doubt that this is a common belief among those who have little knowledge of nutrition science. But let us again consider how the trials are different from natural dietary situations that are measured in observational studies. First and foremost, the positive associations that researchers observed between vitamin E level and dementia in the epidemiological studies occur between *low* dietary intake levels of vitamin E in comparison to levels close to the RDA of 22 IU per day. Compare that with the results of the one trial that examined the effects of a vitamin E supplement on cognitive change according to the baseline dietary levels. Only those participants whose vitamin E levels were at or below 9 IU per day at the beginning of the study showed a positive benefit in cognitive decline. Those with vitamin E levels closer to the RDA experienced no additional benefit of the vitamin E supplement.

The scientific data supporting the positive effects of a strategic diet on preventing cognitive decline and Alzheimer's disease, however, is abundantly clear. Let's move on now to the foods you should eat every day to preserve your mind as well as to support your overall well-being.

CHAPTER 3

Foods for Everyday Eating

As you now know, your brain uses nutrients to form the cells' individual parts, to provide the fuel and build the proteins that it needs to function, and to protect the brain's neurons against injury—and we acquire these nutrients from the foods we eat. As our meals and snacks make their way through the body, they're broken down so that the nutrients can be extracted and absorbed. Some are stored in the fat, liver, muscle, or bone, whereas others are released into the bloodstream and carried directly to organs for immediate use. So when you aim to specifically preserve your mind, your diet should be chock-full not just of any nutrients but of those that we know will most dynamically achieve this goal. As it turns out, the brain needs some nutrients more frequently than others, so we need to consume some foods on a daily basis, whereas others can be eaten weekly.

How did I work this out? When I first began to study nutrition and the brain twenty years ago, I started at the nutrient level because that's where much of the science was focused at the time. The research examined the effects of nutrients on neuron cells and the brain through laboratory and animal studies, and vitamin E was one of the most frequently studied nutrients because of its antioxidant properties.

For this reason, my first studies in nutrition and the brain were of the antioxidant nutrients vitamin E, vitamin C, and beta-carotene. I then moved on to the B vitamins and dietary fats. In those early years of my research, there was a lot of resistance in the medical world to the idea that diet had anything to do with dementia. When to my amazement I found that so many of the nutrients I studied were related to cognitive decline and dementia, I shifted my focus to the food groups that were the biggest contributors to these nutrients.

In this chapter, I'll explore the foods that I've learned should be consumed every day to supply your brain with the nutrients it needs to function at its best. They fall into the categories of leafy green vegetables, other vegetables, whole grains, and vegetable oils. To reap even further benefits to your overall health and to keep things interesting at mealtimes, you'll want to vary the foods you eat within each category.

EVERYDAY FOOD #1: LEAFY GREEN VEGETABLES

Among all the different types of vegetables out there, the leafy green variety has shown to be among the most important for protecting cognitive abilities as we age. Leafy green vegetables are rich in a number of nutrients that are implicated as particularly healthy for the brain—folate, lutein, vitamin E, and beta-carotene among them. The darker the leaves, the greater the source of brain-healthy nutrients. This is because carotenoids and other polyphenolic compounds provide the plant with pigment to protect it from the damaging rays of the sun, and those potent nutrients are now yours for the taking. A number of large studies, including my Chicago studies, have shown that it takes only about one serving a day of leafy green vegetables to slow cognitive decline, so you don't have to eat these at every meal. For example, among the participants of the Memory and Aging Project, those who consumed six or more servings per week of leafy green vegetables had a rate of decline in cognitive abilities equivalent to someone eleven years younger!

These are some of my favorite nutrient-dense leafy green vegetables:

arugula

collard greens

kale

mustard greens

romaine lettuce

spinach

Swiss chard

turnip greens

Many of the nutrients in leafy greens are fat soluble and are best absorbed when they're eaten with a healthy fat such as extra-virgin olive oil, nuts, avocado, or fatty fish. In chapter 10, Laura and I share our favorite recipes with leafy green vegetables in a starring role. This versatile vegetable group can be added to just about any dish—soups, salads, stir-fries, egg dishes, casseroles, smoothies, you name it. I suggest 1 cup of raw leafy greens or ½ cup cooked each day. But if you want to eat more, all the better.

CHEERS TO A HEALTHY BRAIN

If you enjoy a glass of wine with dinner, you'll be heartened to learn that moderate alcohol consumption has an established relation to better cardiovascular health—and there is mounting evidence that this is also true for brain health. Now, when I say moderate consumption, I mean no more than one serving per day for women and two servings per day for men. A serving size is equivalent to 5 ounces of wine, 12 ounces of regular beer (5 percent alcohol), or 1.5 ounces of liquor. Don't go overboard here.

In study after study, the lowest rates of heart attack and dementia are in moderate drinkers compared with those who abstain from alcohol or consume more than one or two drinks per day. Moderate alcohol consumption raises high-density lipoprotein (HDL) cholesterol, the good cholesterol that absorbs bad cholesterol (LDL) and transports it to the liver to be flushed from the body.

It's important to note, however, that with each additional serving over moderate intake, your risk to the heart and brain increases. Heavy alcohol consumption negatively affects every organ of the body, and there is an alcohol-related dementia characterized by impairments in thinking, planning, and memory. Brain-imaging studies have shown greater atrophy of the brain with higher alcohol consumption. Alcohol is addictive, which means your tolerance level increases with more drinks, making it easier to overdo it. Your ability to metabolize alcohol also decreases with age, so the optimal serving for healthy brain and body functioning in old age is actually lower than the one or two servings recommended for younger adults.

EVERYDAY FOOD #2: OTHER VEGETABLES

There are numerous brain-boosting vegetables beyond the leafy green variety. You'll want to include these among the foods you eat every day, too.

Though all the vegetables listed here are teeming with cognitive-enhancing nutrients, cruciferous veggies seem to confer extra special protection to the brain. These include broccoli, bok choy, brussels sprouts, cabbage, and cauliflower. In a study of 13,388 participants of the Nurses' Health Study, those who ate cruciferous vegetables while in their middle-aged years experienced a slower decline in memory, beginning at seventy years old.[25] The Doetinchem Cohort Study conducted in the Netherlands found that eating cabbage was associated with a slower decline in how quickly subjects could think through problems on a regular basis.[26] In my diet study of the Chicago Health and Aging Project, the participants who consumed one or two weekly servings of cruciferous vegetables had slower decline in their thinking abilities overall compared to those who didn't eat these vegetables.[27] The more vegetables you consume, the better off you — and your brain — will be.

Most studies of vegetables and health, including my own, do not include white potatoes as a vegetable. White potatoes are high in many important dietary components, including protein and fiber (about 15 percent and 20 percent of recommended levels, respectively), minerals, and vitamin C. The problem with potatoes is that they have what's known as a "high glycemic index" due to high amounts of simple carbohydrates. The carbs cause blood glucose and insulin levels to spike, which makes you feel hungry again soon after the meal... which then leads to consuming more calories than you need! In combined studies conducted at Harvard of nearly two hundred thousand male and female health professionals, each additional potato serving per day (baked, boiled mashed, or french fried) was associated with a weight gain of 1.3 pounds every four years;[28] seven or more servings of potatoes per week were associated with a 33 percent greater risk of developing type 2 diabetes;[29] and the risk of hypertension was increased by 17 percent for four or more servings of french fries and by 11 percent for four or more servings of baked, boiled, or mashed potatoes.[30] And while there is no data to directly link potato consumption with dementia, there *are* indirect linkages through cardiovascular-related conditions that are known to increase the risk of dementia. Every once in a while, I enjoy baked or mashed potatoes, but they're more of an occasional treat than a regular part of my diet. If potatoes make frequent appearances at your mealtimes, try to replace them with whole-grain bread, brown rice, or another vegetable.

Be mindful about how you prepare your vegetables, including leafy greens. A common misconception is that enjoying them raw is always better for you than eating them cooked. Raw wins out only for only some nutrients; others are actually more bioavailable when they're boiled, steamed, or sautéed. For instance, ½ cup of cooked spinach contains 10,177 micrograms of lutein, 131 micrograms of folate, and 1.34 milligrams of vitamin E—but when it's raw, 1 cup of spinach contains 3,659 micrograms lutein, 36 micrograms of folate, and 0.15 milligrams of vitamin E. So if given the choice, you definitely want to cook your spinach. Fat-soluble nutrients, such as vitamin E and carotenoids, are enhanced rather than reduced when cooked. On the other hand, water-soluble nutrients, such as vitamin C and folate, are leached out of vegetables when they're boiled or steamed, so to absorb these vitamins, raw vegetables are a better source. To capitalize on a healthy intake of all nutrients, I suggest consuming a variety of both raw and cooked vegetables.

Another common misconception about vegetables is that fresh produce has a higher nutritional content than either canned or frozen produce. You might be surprised to know that this is true only if you've picked the vegetable or fruit at its peak growth and then eaten it right away! Most people, however, don't have direct access to their produce's source—and even if they do have a home garden or live on an orchard, they don't time the harvest at peak growth for nutritional value. Commercial produce that you buy at the store is usually picked before its nutritional peak period and increasingly loses its nutrient content with every day after the harvest—during transit, storage, and finally sitting out at the market and then in your refrigerator. Frozen produce, on the other hand, is picked at its peak nutritional value and immediately blanched and frozen to retain its nutrient content up to the time of meal preparation. (*Blanching* is a cooking process by which the fruit or vegetable is first briefly immersed in boiling water and then in ice water to halt the cooking process.) When choosing frozen produce at your local supermarket, try to select packages in which the produce is loose as opposed to frozen together in chunks of ice. The ice chunks indicate that the blanching process was performed in such a way that the nutrient content will not be well preserved.

These are some of my favorite nutrient-dense "other vegetables":

asparagus

beets

broccoli

brussels sprouts

cabbage

carrots

cauliflower

celery

cucumber

eggplant

green beans

leeks

mushrooms

okra

onions

peas

radishes

squash

sweet peppers

sweet potatoes

yams

zucchini

I recommend at least one "other vegetable" serving a day; my diet includes three or four every day. In chapter 11, Laura and I feature some of our best-loved veggie recipes for you to enjoy.

EVERYDAY FOOD #3: WHOLE GRAINS

Unfortunately, whole grains have gotten a bad rap in recent years, but they're rich in brain-healthy minerals and B vitamins and are a moderate source of vitamin E. They're also a great source of fiber, which improves digestion, helps maintain weight, decreases LDL cholesterol, and regulates blood sugar. And while there's almost no scientific investigation into the effects of whole grains or fiber on cognitive decline and dementia, whole grains and fiber *have* been shown to reduce the risk of developing the major cardiovascular risk factors for developing cognitive issues—hypertension, diabetes, obesity, and coronary heart disease.

If you're concerned about, or don't eat, gluten, whole-grain alternatives include corn, rice, sorghum, teff, and some oats. When buying gluten-free oats, look for items that are certified gluten-free because otherwise they might have been contaminated with wheat during their growing or processing. "Pseudo grains" or non-grasses (seeds) are also gluten-free alternatives and include buckwheat, millet, quinoa, and amaranth. They have similar cooking properties and nutritional content to whole grains. Quinoa is especially nutritious, since it's the only plant source that's a complete protein. Most pseudo grains can be cooked in as little as fifteen minutes. Prepared with beans, nuts, and vegetables, they make for quick, tasty, and nutritious meals.

Whole grains include the bran, germ, and endosperm parts of the plant, which are the most dense in nutrients, whereas refined grains are processed to separate the endosperm from the bran and germ before milling, which removes a lot of the grain's nutritional benefits. When buying foods made with grains, check to see that the term "whole grains" is the first ingredient on the label (or the second ingredient after water). But be warned that food manufacturers can label their products—especially breads, cereals, and crackers—as having "whole grains" as long as one serving has at least 8 grams of whole grains. So to cost-effectively bulk up their items, manufacturers use a mix of whole *and* refined grains.

A Harvard School of Public Health study evaluated more than five hundred of these food products and found that those with the highest whole-grain content had at least 1 gram of fiber for every 10 grams of total carbohydrates on the nutrition facts label.[31] How can this help you out? Well, doing the simple math of dividing total carbohydrates by 10 and comparing it to the amount of dietary fiber is a quick way to roughly assess the amount of whole grains in a manufactured food. For instance, if a nutrition label for multigrain crackers says that your total carbohydrates are 24 grams, you'd divide that by 10, which is 2.4 grams. Then, you'd compare it to the dietary fiber amount, which is 3 grams. The fiber content of 3 grams is larger than 2.4 grams, which means the product is mostly whole grain. It's a relief to know, too, that the study found that items with a 10:1 ratio had less added sugar, sodium, and trans fats—a great bonus.

Nutrient-dense whole grains include the following:

buckwheat

brown and wild rice

bulgur

cornmeal

farro

millet

oats

popcorn

quinoa

rye

sorghum

spelt

teff

I suggest three servings of whole grains a day. In chapter 9, you'll find a nice selection of whole-grain dishes to make at home. For other meals, know that according to the US Dietary Guidelines, one serving of whole grains is equivalent to any of these:

½ cup cooked brown rice or other cooked grain

½ cup cooked 100% whole-grain pasta

½ cup cooked hot cereal, such as oatmeal

1 ounce uncooked whole-grain pasta, brown rice, or other grain

1 slice 100% whole-grain bread

1 very small (1 ounce) 100% whole-grain muffin

1 cup 100% whole-grain ready-to-eat cereal

THE CASE FOR WHOLE GRAINS

An extremely popular fad these days is to call for the elimination of whole grains and other foods that contain carbohydrates, including fruits, when aiming to prevent or treat cognitive concerns. For example, Dr. David Perlmutter's hit book *Grain Brain* claims that the cause of Alzheimer's disease is related to grains and carbohydrates. He believes that these dietary components increase inflammation and decrease insulin sensitivity, which causes damage to the brain. It is true that Alzheimer's disease involves inflammation and that impaired insulin sensitivity and glucose metabolism increase the risk of the disease, but this is where the link to the scientific evidence ends with Dr. Perlmutter's hypothesis.

Numerous studies, including dietary intervention trials of diets rich in whole grains, have demonstrated *decreased* inflammation and oxidative stress, *decreased* occurrence of cardiovascular conditions and diseases, and *improved* cognition. For example, the PREDIMED trial that I mentioned in chapter 2 randomly assigned 7,447 people age fifty-five to eighty to one of three diet groups: Mediterranean diet plus olive oil, Mediterranean diet plus nuts, and a low-fat control group (we'll explore the Mediterranean diet in more detail in chapter 6). The purpose of this trial was to test the effects of the Mediterranean diet on the prevention of major cardiovascular events, including heart attack, stroke, and death from heart-related causes. The study participants did not have cardiovascular disease when they were enrolled in the study, but they were at an increased risk of developing it because they had either type 2 diabetes or at least three major risk factors (smoking, hypertension, elevated LDL cholesterol levels, low HDL cholesterol levels, overweight or obesity, or a family history of premature coronary heart disease). Among other foods, both of the Mediterranean diet groups included three or more servings each day of both whole grains and fruits. And sure enough, both experienced a 30 percent decrease in major cardiovascular events.

Cognitive benefits surfaced as well. In 522 of the PREDIMED study participants, performance on cognitive tests was measured after six and a half years on the diet interventions.[32] The Mediterranean diet groups were found to have higher cognitive test scores at the end of the six and a half years compared with the low-fat control group. In another subgroup from this trial, higher consumption of fruits and cereals was associated with lower concentrations of interleukin-6 (IL-6) measured in the serum of participants.[33] IL-6 is a marker of inflammatory and autoimmune processes in many diseases, among them diabetes, atherosclerosis, depression, and Alzheimer's disease.

However, some people cannot consume gluten, present in many grains. The gluten-free diet is an effective therapy for celiac disease, in which the immune system attacks the lining of the small intestine in response to gluten exposure. Gluten is made from different proteins found in wheat and other grains, and damage to the intestinal lining impairs nutrient absorption, causing malnutrition and weight loss. Celiac symptoms include gas, bloating, diarrhea, constipation, headache, trouble concentrating, and fatigue. And while celiac is a genetic disease that affects 1 percent of the population, it's been on the rise in recent years. Even so, a much higher percentage of the population has non-celiac "gluten sensitivity" rather than proper celiac disease. The research on gluten sensitivity is very limited and not consistent enough to verify that it is indeed gluten that causes the symptoms. With little guidance from the scientific community on the topic, I would encourage those who experience food sensitivities to listen to their bodies. Experiment with different whole grains rather than completely eliminating an entire dietary component that has so many documented health benefits and supplies many brain-healthy nutrients.

EVERYDAY FOOD #4: VEGETABLE OILS

Vegetable oils are an important source of what we call healthy fats—that is, monounsaturated and polyunsaturated fats. They're also an excellent source of vitamin E and, for some oil varieties, polyphenols, as in extra-virgin olive oil, and alpha-linolenic acid, a plant-based omega-3 fatty acid in walnut and flaxseed oil. Vitamin E and omega-3 fatty acids are nutrients that have been directly linked to brain health and a lower risk of dementia in scientific studies. Polyphenols are potent antioxidants in plants, but their effect in humans is still not well known. This is a relatively new and exciting field of research.

There is a terrific variety of vegetable oils made from seeds (think olive, canola, sesame) as well as tree nuts (walnut and peanut), each with varying amounts of monounsaturated, polyunsaturated, and saturated fats. The more saturated the fat content, the higher your cooking temperature can go before the oil oxidizes. For this reason, high-heat frying and stir-frying are best with corn, soybean, peanut, and sesame oils. When sautéing over medium-high heat, you should use olive, canola, and grapeseed oils. Finally, save your oils with high omega-3 fatty acid content like flaxseed and walnut oils for salad dressings and dips. To make life easy, I suggest using extra-virgin olive oil as your primary oil. Use 2 tablespoons of it each day, perhaps on a salad or even a slice of bread in place of butter or other spreads. It is also my favorite oil for sautéing spinach and other vegetables. Add a bit of onion and a little garlic — delicious!

Extra-virgin olive oil is an important part of the Mediterranean diet, which means it should be a key part of yours, too. As we saw in the PREDIMED trial, extra-virgin olive oil is thought to have protective effects against dementia by providing a dietary-fat composition with a high ratio of unsaturated to saturated fat, not to mention anti-inflammatory and antioxidant properties.

What makes extra-virgin olive oil so special? It is made from crushed olives and is not refined by chemical solvents or high heat. While the production of high-grade pure oil is expensive since it requires special growing and handling, the refining process that creates a much cheaper product also destroys polyphenols through oxidation. Unfortunately, much of the olive oil out there that's labeled "extra-virgin" is in fact adulterated with refined oil or otherwise low-standard production practices. No wonder there's a huge black market for olive oil, especially from Italy. The industry isn't regulated, so just because the label on a bottle says your olive oil was imported from Italy, this doesn't guarantee that it's a high-quality extra-virgin olive oil. To be sure that your oil is as good as it gets, look for certification seals by national and state olive oil associations, such as the Australian Olive Association, the California Olive Oil Council (COOC), the Italian Agricultural Confederation (CIA), and the Association 3E. The COOC, for example, certifies California oils every growing season. To receive a seal of approval for "extra-virgin," the oil has to come from perfectly ripened olives that are milled within twenty-four hours of harvest. It also can't be chemically treated and must pass numerous chemical tests. In addition, COOC certification includes taste tests to ensure that the oil has peppery, fruity, and bitter flavors and no hint of vinegar or rancidness.

These are among the most nutrient-dense vegetable oils:

canola (rapeseed)

corn

cottonseed

grapeseed

olive

peanut

safflower

sesame

soybean

sunflower

walnut

A WORD ABOUT COCONUT OIL

While we're talking oil, I'm frequently asked about the brain-health benefits of coconut oil. There's currently limited scientific data to back up the claims that it has therapeutic effects in Alzheimer's disease patients. This could change, however, with the conclusion of a randomized controlled trial that is currently underway.

Coconut oil comes from the coconut fruit and contains high levels of saturated fat (about 84 percent of its total calories, compared with 63 percent in butter). Its health benefits for Alzheimer's patients are believed to come from medium-chain fatty acids that are easily absorbed and metabolized by the liver. These can then be converted to ketones, which are an alternative to glucose energy in the brain. In Alzheimer's disease the glucose uptake into neurons is impaired, so medium-chain fatty acids are thought to be of benefit. A few clinical studies have also shown that coconut oil increases fat burning, reduces abdominal fat, and has favorable effects on blood cholesterol, which has caused some to postulate that it could be helpful for diabetes and heart disease. However, other clinical studies demonstrate unfavorable effects on blood cholesterol and glucose. The current research on coconut oil's health benefits is just too limited for me to suggest you eat it for mind preservation.

Are you as hungry as I am right now for a bowl of hearty grains, tossed with fresh veggies and extra-virgin olive oil? How about a glass of red wine on the side? Great! Then my job here is done. Next up: foods you'll want to eat every week for a strong and nimble mind.

CHAPTER 4

Foods to Eat Every Week

To understand why certain foods need to be eaten every day and others at various frequencies every week, it's helpful to take a look at why we began studying nutrition's relationship to disease patterns at all

Though research on the links between diet and illness is constantly evolving, believe it or not, we've been at this for a long time. In fact, researchers have been studying diet patterns since the mid-1900s! As I mentioned in the last chapter, nutrition science used to focus more on how nutrients and nutrient deficiencies impacted disease. It wasn't until the 1960s that we began examining death rates by country and found that those who lived in the regions around the Mediterranean Sea—particularly in Greece and southern Italy—had some of the longest life expectancies in the world. They also had very low rates of heart disease, certain cancers, and other chronic illnesses that we associate with aging. This, despite the fact that modern healthcare wasn't as available there as it was in more westernized parts of the world.

Such significant observations spurred additional studies that described, in detail, the diet of Mediterranean cultures. They studied how different diet patterns (say, Mediterranean versus westernized diets) affected the development of chronic illnesses like heart disease and diabetes. They also tracked whether eating certain food groups (like seafood and meats) played a role in these conditions. In my own research, once it became clear that nutrition had a lot to do with brain health, I began to investigate nutrition and dementia and cognitive decline in the same way, and my discoveries fill this chapter. It's no coincidence that many of the foods here are common among Mediterranean diets, too.

In the previous chapter, we focused on food groups that satisfy the daily nutritional needs of the brain; here, I'll focus on weekly suggestions that should be folded into your diet. This doesn't mean that these nutrients are less important; your brain simply doesn't need them replenished in the same frequency or amount. In fact, with some foods, like seafood, more is not necessarily shown to do more for you. But these are healthy foods, so if you like to eat them more often, feel free to do so. Just be careful that you do not take in more calories than you expend through physical activity so that you maintain a healthy weight—this is very easy to do with nuts, for example. I'll also explain how different servings of berries, nuts, seafood, poultry, and legumes supply your brain with the tocopherols, B vitamins, folate, healthy fats, carotenoids, and polyphenols that are needed to protect the brain from oxidative stress, inflammation, and DNA damage. Some of these nutrients have also been found to improve vascular function, synaptic transmission, and neuronal function to help your brain and heart work as one.

EVERY WEEK FOOD #1: BERRIES

I love berries! They are one of my favorite foods because they taste so good. It is sheer bonus that they are also packed with antioxidants and phytochemicals, and are so easy to eat. Just a quick rinse and they are ready to take on the go. They can be added to cereal, yogurt, or salads, eaten alone as a snack, or whirled into smoothies. One of my favorite breakfasts is warm Blueberry-Apple Pancakes (page 143). It takes no time to make and is delicious and healthy, too!

Much of what we know about the remarkable impact of berries on brain health comes from animal models in which extraordinary effects were observed for blueberries, strawberries, blackberries, and cranberries. In aged rodents, blueberry and strawberry extracts either attenuated or reversed both motor and cognitive functioning deficits.[34] The mice experienced better memory skills, and the hippocampal region of their brains, which is key for memory function, actually generated new neurons. Remember, too, that the hippocampus is where we know Alzheimer's disease begins.

A few large epidemiological studies, including my own investigations of older Chicagoan residents, confirm the extensive research that's been conducted in animals. In these human studies, subjects who ate berries at least once a week had a significantly slower decline in cognitive abilities. And in the largest research study to date, blueberry and strawberry consumption during midlife was measured in 16,010 women of the Nurses' Health Study and related to their decline in cognitive abilities during their 70s.[35] Compared with the nurses who consumed blueberries less than once per month, those who consumed one or more servings of the berries on a weekly basis had slower rates of cognitive decline. What's more, this was after taking into account other factors associated with better cognitive functioning, like education, income, and physical exercise. Similar findings were observed for the nurses who consumed two or more servings of strawberries per week. The authors of the study concluded that cognitive aging was delayed by up to 2.5 years among women with higher blueberry and strawberry intakes. In other investigations of these same nurses, eating two or more servings a week of berries was associated with 24 percent greater odds of aging healthfully — more specifically, these nurses had no major chronic diseases or major impairments in their thinking abilities, physical function, or mental health.[36]

In my two Chicago studies, those who ate berries experienced cognitive decline at the pace of someone who was two to six years younger — this in 3,768 CHAP participants age sixty-five and older, and in 959 of the much older MAP participants. In addition, among the MAP participants who were free of dementia at the beginning of the study, those who ate two or more servings of berries each week were 52 percent less likely to develop Alzheimer's disease over an average period of five years!

These promising findings are supported by a 2017 randomized trial in humans in which both the investigators and the participants were blinded to the type of berry intervention they were receiving, either a freeze-dried blueberry equivalent to 1 cup of fresh blueberries or a blueberry placebo. After just ninety days of the intervention, the participants in the blueberry group showed significantly fewer errors in tests of learning.[37]

Berries get their brain-healthy superpowers from carotenoids and flavonoids, two classes of phytochemicals with potent antioxidant and anti-inflammatory properties. Blueberries are particularly rich in the flavonoid anthocyanin, which is where the purple and red colors of plants come from. It's actually the skin, rather than the fruit flesh, that gives us this phytochemical. Among other foods that contain high amounts of anthocyanins are cherries (122 milligrams anthocyanin per 100 grams cherries), blood oranges (200 milligrams/100 grams), acai (320 milligrams/100 grams), Concord grapes (326 milligrams/100 grams), eggplant (750 milligrams/100 grams), and purple corn (1,642 milligrams/100 grams).

Anthocyanins have promising implications for Alzheimer's disease.

In the study of rodents I mentioned previously, those that were fed blueberry extract had increased levels of anthocyanin in the hippocampal region of the brain. Remarkably, these levels were correlated directly with increases in cognitive performance, which strongly implicates anthocyanin as an important dietary component in neurogenesis and memory performance. In other words, eating blueberries may improve memory function through the growth of neurons in the brain's memory region. This has not been examined in the human brain as of yet.

It's important to mention, too, that unlike frozen vegetables, frozen berries are processed in a way that can impact their nutrient count — specifically, their flavonoid content. For instance, 100 grams of frozen raspberries (approximately ¾ cup) contain 24 milligrams of anthocyanins, or half the anthocyanin content found in fresh raspberries (48 milligrams). Similarly, frozen blueberries provide 94 milligrams anthocyanins versus 163 in fresh berries. Cooking will also decrease a berry's anthocyanin levels.

So, based on these animal and human studies, I suggest eating at least 1 cup of berries every week. The fresher, the better! Berry recipes are sprinkled throughout part II of this book, since they can be both a versatile accent and a main attraction.

These are my favorite nutrient-dense berries:

acai berries

blackberries

blueberries

cranberries

raspberries

strawberries

WHAT ABOUT OTHER FRUIT?

Though other types of fruit have substantial levels of flavonoids and carotenoids and have been linked to lower risks of cancer, osteoporosis, and cardiovascular diseases, they have not been associated with protecting against brain-related aging and neuro-degenerative disease. In fact, five large epidemiological studies investigated the relationship between the two, and no associations were found. Oranges, for instance, have high levels of fla-vonols but don't slow cognitive decline. Yet because fruits are potent antioxidant and fiber sources that may benefit the rest of your body, I do believe they should be part of your diet. Many fruits are high in calories, so just be sure not to overconsume.

EVERY WEEK FOOD #2: NUTS

Nuts are an excellent source of many brain-healthy nutrients, including vitamin E, B vitamins, and healthy fats—each nut with its own levels of goodness. For example, 1 ounce of almonds provides about half of the recommended daily allowance of alpha tocopherol (vitamin E), whereas walnuts, pistachios, and pecans are excellent sources of gamma tocopherol. In chapter 2, I described how gamma tocopherol has anti-inflammatory and antioxidant properties and may be important for dementia prevention. Peanuts (which are botanically legumes but nutritionally considered a nut), the most-consumed nut in the United States, are a good source of protein (1 ounce provides about 15 percent of the RDA for women and 13 percent for men) and folate (1 ounce contains 17 percent of the RDA). Nuts also have a higher ratio of polyunsaturated and monounsaturated fats to saturated fats compared with many other foods.

If you had to pick a winner for brain-enhancing nuts, walnuts would take first prize. They are one of the nuts highest in gamma tocopherol, and they have the highest composition of polyunsaturated fatty acids, including alpha linolenic acid. In fact, of all the edible plants, walnuts have the highest content of this essential omega-3 fatty acid. In animal studies done at Tufts University, rodents fed the equivalent of about 1 ounce of walnuts a day performed better on learning and memory tests.[38] Walnuts were also part of the Mediterranean diet in the Spanish PREDIMED randomized trial that demonstrated better performance on cognitive ability tests.

Nuts influence the healthy brain and heart crossover effect, too. In multiple large studies on nuts and cardiovascular disease, including the PREDIMED trial, two to five servings of this brain food per week were associated with 37 percent fewer deaths from coronary heart disease. Such a reduced risk may be due in part to how nuts improve blood cholesterol. In multiple human studies, eating nuts decreased both LDL and total cholesterol. One type of compound contained in nuts, called phytosterols, may be partly responsible for their ability to lower cholesterol, since phytosterols compete with the body's ability to absorb cholesterol from food.

For maximum brain-enhancing advantages, eat 1 ounce, or about a handful, of a variety of nuts two to five times a week. However, be careful not to overdo it. Nuts are also high in calories — for example, 1 ounce of peanuts has 161 calories. I recommend low-salt or unsalted nuts, as higher sodium increases your blood pressure and hypertension, a primary risk factor for stroke. I'm a big fan of nuts as an afternoon or post-workout snack or sprinkled on a salad. However, because I find it hard to keep to just a 1-ounce serving (nuts are addictive!), lately I have started to restrict my nut intake to a garnish on my salads. Otherwise, I tend to take in many more calories than is good for controlling my weight.

Here are some of my favorite nutrient-dense nuts:

almonds

Brazil nuts

cashews

macadamia nuts

peanuts

pecans

pistachio nuts

walnuts

IS CHOCOLATE A BRAIN FOOD?

As early as the seventeenth century, chocolate and cocoa were used to medically treat angina and heart pain. And in recent years, very promising research supports the benefits of cocoa on heart health, as well as inflammatory bowel disease, cancer, and the brain. There are more than three hundred biologically active compounds in cocoa, including flavonoids (such as catechins) and other polyphenolic compounds. In fact, cocoa powder and dark chocolate rank among the top food sources for polyphenolic content and antioxidant capacity, measuring twice as high as green tea or red wine and four to five times higher than black tea.

As for its effects on mental faculties, a number of small clinical trials have shown that cocoa is effective in increasing blood flow to the brain and resistance to oxidative stress; decreasing blood pressure and blood clotting; and improving the blood cholesterol profile and blood sugar regulation. For all these reasons, it's possible that cocoa may be protective against the brain's aging process. In fact, one randomized trial of older adults found that a dairy-based cocoa drink consumed daily for eight weeks resulted in higher performance on cognitive tests compared to adults who drank a placebo.[39] Even though these studies are promising, I do not think that the scientific evidence on the brain effects of cocoa-derived foods is yet at a level to recommend them for brain health. The randomized trials are small, of short duration, and mostly supported by the food industry, which can benefit from the results of the studies. In addition, the cocoa products used in these trials are different from the products available to consumers — they contain much higher levels of polyphenolic compounds. When cocoa beans are processed to make foods, their flavonoid content is significantly reduced. Better processing techniques need to be developed to preserve the polyphenols in cocoa-based products, and large randomized controlled trials need to be conducted that are not industry sponsored.

EVERY WEEK FOOD #3: SEAFOOD

When some people hear that eating seafood can help their brains become more resilient to aging and cognitive decline, their first instinct is to take pause — *Do I have to eat it every night? Is it going to get expensive? What about mercury and other toxins?* If this is you, I'm about to put your worries to rest. And if it isn't, that's even better! Seafood is incredibly beneficial to the brain. In addition to the favorable effects that I described in earlier chapters, the omega-3 fatty acids in seafood are key to a healthy cardiovascular system that supplies blood and nutrients to the brain. Omega-3s regulate the beating of the heart and help prevent fatal erratic rhythms. They also lower blood pressure through their effects on the contraction and relaxation of artery walls, and they lower triglyceride levels, which play a role in the development of atherosclerosis. There are so many studies that demonstrate the beneficial effects of these fats on cardiovascular disease that the American Heart Association recommends eating two 3- to 5-ounce servings of seafood a week.

Many studies around the world have examined the relationship between seafood and dementia, and the results aren't just consistent; they're exceptional and find a significant, lower risk *with just one seafood meal per week*. Yes, just one! This has even been demonstrated in a study of non-industrialized countries,[40] including Cuba, the Dominican Republic, Mexico, Peru, and China—an important finding because seafood consumption in nonindustrialized countries is often associated with lower socioeconomic status, which is also a risk factor for dementia. And if you want to feast on seafood more than once a week, have at it. There aren't any health detriments to eating fish more frequently. I happen to love fish, so I consume three or more servings per week. Just know that there's little scientific evidence that more fish offers more benefits. Laura and I have filled chapter 13 to the gills with wonderful seafood recipes that family and guests will love.

What About Contaminants?

Over the years, the mercury content in fish has been a concern. So, in our study of nearly one thousand participants of the Chicago Memory and Aging Project, we examined the brain tissue of 203 participants who died over the course of the study, looking for high mercury levels.[41] Even though we noticed a small positive correlation between the brain levels of mercury and the amount of fish these participants ate during their later years of life, the mercury levels were not associated with increases in brain neuropathologies.

Furthermore, those participants who consumed one or more seafood meals per week had *lower* accumulation of the Alzheimer's disease neuropathologies — both the amyloid beta plaques and the neurofibrillary tangles. Eating one or more seafood meals a week was also associated with slower cognitive decline in 994 of the MAP participants whose cognitive abilities were tested on an annual basis for up to ten years.[42] A few other studies that measured mercury levels in blood tissue also found no association with cognitive function in older adults. It should be noted, however, that mercury exposure to developing fetuses, infants, and children up to adolescence may pose health risks and should be avoided. Mercury and other toxic chemicals can disrupt a child's developing brain and immune system and affect learning and behavior. Pediatric experts recommend that expectant mothers and children consume fish to get the health benefits but choose fish that is low in mercury. The Environmental Protection Agency and the US Food and Drug Administration (FDA) provide online advice on what fish to eat for pregnant women and parents (see www.fda.gov/Food/Foodborne IllnessContaminants/Metals/ucm393070.htm).

If you're a seafood lover, you'll be pleased to know that mercury levels are actually declining in the environment. The seafood with the highest levels of mercury are at the top of the food chain and have been around the longest period of time to accumulate toxins. Therefore, pregnant women and others who wish to limit their mercury exposure should avoid marlin, shark, swordfish, tilefish, orange roughy, and bluefin tuna. Canned light tuna is among the safest fish to eat in terms of mercury exposure. In a study conducted by the University of Nevada, Las Vegas, mercury levels in canned light tuna were found to be three times lower than those in canned white (albacore) tuna.[43] Other fish that are safe to eat according to the FDA include salmon, catfish, flounder, sole, trout, black sea bass, tilapia, pollock, anchovies, herring, and perch. Shellfish such as oysters, shrimp, crab, clams, and scallops are also low in mercury. It should be noted that whereas early studies reported higher levels of PCBs (polychlorinated biphenyls) and other contaminants in farmed salmon compared with ocean or wild fish, more recent investigations have not confirmed this, and the consensus is that both farmed and wild salmon are safe to eat. Studies have also shown that the levels of omega-3 fatty acids in farmed salmon are similar to those of wild or ocean species because the fish are now given feeds containing omega-3s.

Fish consumption can also increase your exposure to toxins other than mercury, including PCBs, PBDEs (polybrominated diphenyl ethers), dioxins, and chlorinated pesticides, though how you prepare and cook your fish will minimize this concern — especially with pollutants like PCBs and pesticides that concentrate in fish fat. These toxins wind up in streams, rivers, lakes, and oceans through industrial and municipal discharges, agricultural practices, and storm-water runoff. To reduce your exposure by 50 percent, remove the fish's skin and fat before cooking it and try broiling, grilling, or baking, since fat drips off the fish through these means. Just know that these tricks won't cut mercury contamination, since mercury is stored in the meat of the fish as opposed to the fat. To date there have been almost no informative studies on the effects of toxins other than mercury on dementia and cognitive decline.

There are many people out there who simply don't like fish and ask me if they can get the same brain benefit by eating plant sources of the omega-3 fatty acid alpha linolenic acid (ALA), found in flaxseed, chia seeds, walnuts, and canola oil. The honest answer is that we don't know. The scientific evidence is just too limited to make any claims with confidence about the effects that ALA plant sources have on the brain. Humans can convert ALA to the longer-chain omega-3 fatty acids DHA and EPA, but the conversion rate is less than 1 percent. Whether this is sufficient to supply the brain with the level of DHA required to function optimally with older age isn't clear. In my study of dietary omega-3 fatty acids and the brain in the Memory and Aging Project, we did find evidence that dietary intake of ALA was associated with a slower decline in cognitive abilities and less stroke pathologies in the brain. Yet the evidence for ALA and dementia across a number of other epidemiological studies is not at all consistent; this may be due to the difficulty of accurately measuring the nutrient's intake and absorption.

People also ask if they can take fish oil supplements rather than eat fish. Visit any vitamin shop and there are so many versions to choose from that you might assume this was based on strong scientific evidence. Several randomized clinical trials have been conducted to investigate whether DHA and EPA supplements can reduce cognitive decline in older adults. Yet overall, study results have not been positive, though there has been some evidence of beneficial effects in subgroups of individuals, such as those who have a specific genotype, or those with little evidence of mild cognitive impairment. The lack of consistency in these trials' findings tells me that there is a lot that we don't understand about the metabolism of omega-3 fatty acids and their impact on the human brain.

These are some of the more nutrient-dense seafood options:

herring

lake trout

oysters

Pacific chub mackerel

pollock

salmon

sardines

scallops

sea bass

shrimp

squid

tuna (fresh ahi tuna and canned light tuna)

EVERY WEEK FOOD #4: POULTRY

If you're a fan of poultry, then you're in for good news. While there is no direct evidence in the scientific literature that links poultry to nutrition and the brain, I do recommend making it part of your weekly diet, with two or more 3- to 5-ounce servings per week. To help you judge serving sizes, a 3-ounce portion is equivalent to one split chicken breast or chicken leg (drumstick plus thigh).

Here's why: First, this recommended serving of poultry is roughly equivalent to that of the DASH and Mediterranean diets, two diets we'll discuss in more detail in chapter 6 that have been rigorously tested and found to prevent many cardiovascular-related diseases and conditions. As I describe in chapter 1, heart-healthy diets are good for the brain. Second, poultry is an excellent, low-fat source of B vitamins, a class of nutrients that is important for maintaining brain health. Poultry is also a source of tryptophan, an essential amino acid that acts as a building block in the making of proteins essential for us to live. (Some examples of great nonmeat sources of tryptophan include soybeans, egg whites, and sesame and sunflower seeds.) The B vitamin niacin (B_3) is synthesized from tryptophan, too. In the Chicago Health and Aging Project, we found that eating foods that contain both niacin and tryptophan was associated with slower rates of cognitive decline and the risk of developing Alzheimer's disease.[44] To my knowledge, this finding has not been investigated by other studies and therefore shouldn't be taken as confirmed evidence that niacin prevents Alzheimer's disease or cognitive decline, but it is promising data.

Niacin supplementation is often used along with statin drugs in the treatment of heart disease thanks to its positive effects on blood cholesterol and triglycerides—and a healthy cholesterol profile points to one possible mechanism by which dietary intake of niacin may be beneficial to the brain. Even so, there is a lot we don't understand about niacin's effect on brain function. For example, the disease pellagra, caused by niacin deficiency, is characterized by diarrhea, dermatitis, and dementia. The exact mechanisms by which pellagra causes dementia are not known. The disease was once endemic to populations where the staple food was maize untreated by lime, an important process that makes the niacin nutritionally available. Pellagra also occurs in alcoholics, prisoners, and other groups who have severely restricted diets or malabsorption issues. However, niacin supplementation should be monitored by a doctor, due to its possible adverse effects on the liver and glucose metabolism. It may also cause gastrointestinal problems.

In addition to niacin and protein synthesis, tryptophan is key to the synthesis of neurotransmitters in the brain, including serotonin and melatonin. Serotonin regulates sleep, appetite, and mood but is also involved in memory and learning function. Melatonin is known as an important hormone for sleep regulation but also has antioxidant properties. Serotonin, in particular, is being investigated as a factor in the progression of many neurodegenerative diseases, including Alzheimer's disease.

The healthiest way to eat poultry is without the skin and not fried — that is, boiled, baked, or grilled. Also, watch the fat on your poultry. If you're roasting a chicken or turkey, it's best to leave the skin on during the roasting process to keep the meat moist; but be sure to remove it before you carve and serve it since the skin contains a lot of saturated fat. In fact, a roasted chicken breast with the skin has about twice the amount of total and saturated fat as a chicken breast without the skin. Dark meat has slightly more than twice the fat of light meat, but otherwise it's nutritionally equivalent. And game birds, like duck, quail, and pheasant, have about three times the amount of fat found in chicken or turkey.

One easy way to reduce the amount of red meat in your diet is to replace it in casseroles and burgers with ground turkey or chicken. This was how I gradually reduced the amount of red meat that my husband ate. Over a few years, I completely eliminated ground beef from our family meals with no complaints! You'll find some delicious poultry recipes in chapter 13 of this book for your loved ones to savor, too.

EVERY WEEK FOOD #5: BEANS AND OTHER LEGUMES

For centuries, beans and other legumes were the main source of protein in our diets instead of meat. In fact, many traditional vegetarian diets still include filling combinations of lentils and rice, bread and hummus or tahini, and beans with potatoes. The traditional Mediterranean diet, such as the Greek diet in the 1950s, was made up of three to four servings of legumes per week, including beans, lentils, chickpeas, peas, flat beans, and split peas. Beans are an excellent, low-fat source of protein and B vitamins, and therefore an ideal substitute for red meat. Unlike meat, they are also one of the highest food sources of fiber, a dietary component that lowers the risk of cardiovascular conditions shown to increase risk of dementia. There are numerous ways to incorporate beans into your diet — in chili or soups, on salads, in tacos or burritos, in rice or pasta dishes, or as a side dish. In our family, we have both meat eaters and vegetarians. It's easy to accommodate both by, for instance, adding ground turkey to one half of a lasagna dish or soup recipe and beans to the other half, or by preparing both bean and meat fillings for a taco dinner.

Although animal foods like meat, seafood, poultry, and eggs provide the most complete protein for our biological needs, it is a common myth that vegetarians lack adequate protein in their diets. Some vegetable sources of protein contain all the essential amino acids — the basic structural components of protein — but many are lower in one or more of the nine essential amino acids, particularly lysine. A daily vegetarian diet that includes grains and vegetables in addition to legumes produces the "high biological value proteins" that are found in animal foods. You do not need to consume these complementary protein foods in the same meal to obtain optimal nutritional benefits from protein. Try to eat at least four ½-cup servings of legumes every week. You'll find great recipes in chapter 12.

These are some of my favorite nutrient-dense legumes:

beans (black beans, chickpeas, kidney beans, pinto beans, white beans)

edamame (soybeans)

lentils

lima beans

tofu

Now that I've armed you with all the foods you need for a healthy brain—fresh vegetables, hearty whole grains, nourishing vegetable oils, fresh berries, earthy nuts and beans, and brain-boosting seafood—we'll explore the foods that *won't* do your brain any favors. You don't have to swear off them forever; just limit their role in your diet, and you'll be glad you did.

CHAPTER 5

Brainless Foods That Harm the Mind

What I call "brainless foods" are those that contribute to a high intake of saturated and trans fats, simple sugars, salt, and pathogenic compounds called advanced glycation end products. If your diet is riddled with these elements, you're at a higher risk for cardiovascular diseases and diabetes, which also increase your odds of getting dementia. Studies show that saturated and trans fats accelerate cognitive decline and increase the risk of developing dementia *independent of* cardiovascular factors. They're used in the food industry to improve shelf life, food texture, and taste, but they're also a factor in the rising levels of illness in the United States and the world at large.

Before you roll your eyes or put down this book, rest assured that I'm not going to tell you to eliminate all brainless foods from your diet. It's okay to have an occasional sweet or salty treat that you really enjoy, and in chapter 15, we've included snack and dessert recipes that will actually help your brain rather than hurt it the way brainless foods do. So I do endorse guilty pleasures—I have them, too. I don't want you to swear off them altogether and "be good" in the short term but then give up on a healthier diet for life. I also understand that if a food you eat is very high in bad fats, salt, and/or sugar, it may take a considerable amount of time and effort to follow the recommended servings outlined in this book. You *can* do this, though, because your taste buds and food satisfaction can be trained to prefer healthier choices.

Changes in lifestyle behaviors aren't easy, but they're simplest to achieve if you concentrate on them one at a time. It might be a good idea to add the food categories I've mentioned in the previous chapters individually, and over time—and nix the brainless foods in a similar way. If your weakness is to eat dessert every night of the week or a pastry every morning, start by limiting your treat to just five days out of the week instead of seven. You may find that you enjoy it more and look forward to the special treat days. An alternative strategy would be to eat your treat every day but cut each serving in half. Either way, once you've mastered this small change, you can move on to the next one. Before you know it, you'll have a healthier diet and will likely notice your weight, blood pressure, blood cholesterol, and glucose dropping, too. Your body will feel good, and you'll feel proud that you overcame the seemingly impossible.

When I first met my husband, who was tall and slender with a naturally high metabolism, he ate a lot of red meat and high-fat animal products like whole milk and butter. When I first tried to modify his diet, he met my good intentions with contempt and distrust. I'd serve him a meal with a small amount of meat, and he'd look at me as if I was trying to starve him or, at the very least, serve him a "poor man's" diet! Having been raised as a skinny boy with a huge appetite, he was used to being fed a lot of meat, butter, and high-fat dairy. His mom and all his friends' moms were doing their best to fatten him up! I resorted to making very small, gradual changes in his diet, perhaps a little on the sly, such as switching from whole milk to 2 percent and then to skim, mixing higher and higher proportions of ground turkey to ground beef in meatballs or loafs, replacing meat-centric meals with casseroles that had a lot more vegetables and grains, and replacing butter with trans fat–free margarine and extra-virgin olive oil. Fifteen years later, he was the primary cook in our household, making colorful meals that were highly nutritious, balanced, and mostly vegetarian. His culinary skills were a major influence on our health-savvy daughter, Laura, whose delicious recipes appear in part II.

In this chapter, I'll discuss the brainless foods that, if not curbed, will wreak havoc on your health—and, specifically, your brain. A few of them may surprise you.

BRAINLESS FOOD #1: RED MEAT

In recent years, red meat seems to have made a comeback in certain nutrition circles, thanks in part to diet trends like the Paleo diet and the growing popularity of grass-fed beef, purported to have health benefits. Yet for a healthy brain, my long-term research has shown that it's best to limit how much red meat you eat to no more than three 3- to 5-ounce servings a week (a petite woman should eat closer to 3 ounces; a muscular man closer to 5 ounces). This serving size includes the meat you eat with breakfast and on sandwiches, too. To many Americans, this might sound restrictive, but it's worth mentioning that in the traditional Mediterranean diet, meat was reserved for special occasions and eaten no more than once a week. A lot of my concern about meat is the saturated fat, so you can cut this by choosing the leanest cuts, cooking with racks and drip trays to eliminate fat drippings, and trimming any visible fat before cooking and again before eating. Take broiled beef tenderloin, for instance. A little more than a single 3-ounce serving (100 grams) contains 17.1 grams of total fat and 6.7 grams of saturated fat when the meat is trimmed to ⅛ inch of visible fat. But when you trim the visible fat away entirely, you'll have only .7.2 grams of total fat and 3.0 grams of saturated fat left on the meat — *less than half* of the fat that could affect your brain function.

All heart-healthy diets suggest that you limit the amount of red meat you eat, so it's based on this that I suggest limiting red meat consumption to protect your brain. Currently, there is very limited research on how eating meat affects brain health. There is indirect evidence, however, through the positive benefits on cognitive decline and dementia risk with higher adherence to the DASH and Mediterranean diets, given that both diets limit red meat. We'll explore these diets further in the next chapter.

BRAINLESS FOOD #2: DAIRY PRODUCTS AND EGGS

Whole-Fat Cheese

Here in the United States, we have a destructive love affair with cheese that over time may influence how likely you are to experience cognitive decline. In fact, cheese and pizza have surpassed meat as the primary sources of saturated fat in Americans' diet. Cheese contains more fat than you're probably aware of — a 1-ounce serving of American cheese has more saturated fat (5.1 grams) than a serving of lean roast beef (3.4 grams) and almost as much as a broiled beef tenderloin (6.7 grams). In 2015, the annual per capita consumption of cheese in the United States was 33.9 pounds, a 239 percent increase over consumption levels in 1975!

By far, the leading cheeses consumed in the United States are cheddar and mozzarella—the latter of which is likely related to how much pizza we eat. According to a 2014 US Department of Agriculture Food Survey Research Group report, one in eight Americans eats pizza on any given day, providing about a quarter of a person's daily calorie intake! Pizza also ranks as one of the top three contributors to sodium intake among Americans. Pizza made in the United States—unlike pizza in many other countries—is *loaded* with cheese. When making your own pizza, try to use creative ways to reduce the amount and type of cheese you use, including low-fat varieties.

I get it: cheese is delicious, and I'm a bona fide cheese lover myself. But to preserve my brain, I've had to change my way of thinking about the role of cheese in my diet—from that of a major daily player to an accent on a meal or an occasional treat. I rarely eat pizza anymore, nor do I snack on cheese and crackers at lunch or before dinner as I used to do. I try to limit my weekly cheese consumption to a scant tablespoon of feta or goat cheese added to my salads. Otherwise, I indulge only on special occasions. One of my favorite comfort foods is a grilled cheddar cheese sandwich, which I've modified by using less than 1 ounce of cheese layered between onions and/or mushrooms, plus spinach that's been sautéed in extra-virgin olive oil. This allows me to get that grilled cheese flavor but with the healthy addition of the vegetables. And it is delicious! A realistic goal is to limit whole-fat cheese intake to 1 to 2 ounces per week; a 1-ounce serving of hard cheese is about the size of your thumb or 2 tablespoons of crumbled cheese.

In the following table, you'll find the saturated and total fat contents of the most common cheeses eaten in the United States. The harder cheeses — cheddar, Colby, Swiss — are at the top of the list in terms of saturated fat content. When preparing casseroles, consider replacing whole-fat with low-fat cheeses. You'd be surprised at how little the taste or texture changes, and you can cut the fat content considerably. For example, using part-skim mozzarella cheese reduces the saturated fat over the whole-fat varieties by 20 percent, and part-skim ricotta cheese by 40 percent. I often use low-fat cottage cheese (which contains only 0.7 grams of saturated fat per ½ cup) in place of ricotta (10.3 grams saturated fat per ½ cup) in lasagna.

Protein and Fat Content of 1 ounce of Various Cheeses			
Cheese	Protein (g)	Saturated Fat (g)	Total Fat (g)
Cheddar	6.5	5.3	9.4
Colby	6.7	5.7	9.1
Swiss	7.6	5.2	8.8
American	5.1	5.1	8.6
Goat	6.1	5.8	8.5
Blue	6.1	5.3	8.1
Gouda	7.1	5.0	7.8
Brie	5.9	4.9	7.8
Mozzarella	6.3	3.7	6.3
Feta	4.0	4.2	6.0

United States Department of Agriculture, National Agricultural Library. https://ndb.nal .usda.gov/ndb/search

Butter and Stick Margarine

Butter and stick margarine are potent sources of saturated and trans fats, so they should be eaten infrequently — less than one pat per day (about 1½ teaspoons). Butter has a high density of saturated fat: one pat has 4 grams of total fat, of which 2.6 grams (65 percent) is saturated. Many stick margarines contain trans fats and are formed by partially hydrogenating vegetable oils, a chemical process that adds hydrogen to vegetable oils, which are liquid at room temperature, to make them solid. There are plenty of new margarines on the market that do not contain trans fats; these generally come in a tub and should be used in place of butter. An even better alternative is to use olive oil in place of butter or margarine.

Other Dairy

It is worth mentioning other dairy products, although in general there's no direct research on their effects on the brain or on dementia risk. However, because dairy products can be a significant source of saturated fat, I suggest low-fat milk and yogurt.

Eggs

Eggs are in their own special category and deserve a little more explanation. Although eggs are not dairy products, since they come from chickens and not from cows, many people think of them as such because they are sold in the dairy aisle at the supermarket. Eggs have gotten a bad rap in the nutrition world, mainly due to their high cholesterol count. A single large egg contains 186 milligrams of dietary cholesterol. Yet it also contains a significant amount of the daily requirement for vitamin B_{12} (28 percent) and protein (about 10 percent). The yolk of the egg is nutrient dense and contains folate, vitamin D, vitamin E, and lutein. A commonly held belief is that dietary cholesterol is an important factor in raising LDL blood cholesterol, but in fact the most important contributors are saturated and trans fats. Only a small percentage of the population is hyper-responsive to dietary cholesterol. For most of us, then, eating an egg a day, or even seven a week, poses no health risk. Eggs become brainless, however, for people with heart disease or diabetes; they shouldn't eat more than three egg yolks a week. Watch, too, what you eat with your eggs! It would be a terrible idea for your brain, for instance, to smother your omelet with cheese or to eat your eggs with bacon or sausage and white toast.

Even if you have a weakness for eggs, there's been a great deal of research on ways to improve your cholesterol profile. Reducing saturated fat to less than 7 percent of calories will result in an 8 to 10 percent reduction in LDL cholesterol. By comparison, decreasing your dietary cholesterol to less than 200 milligrams per day reduces LDL cholesterol level by only 3 to 5 percent. In total, for many people, dietary changes can reduce LDL cholesterol by 20 to 30 percent, an effect comparable to that of cholesterol-lowering drugs. Rather than give up eggs entirely, you may try other effective dietary strategies for lowering cholesterol like losing weight and increasing the amount of vegetables, fruits, cereals, legumes, vegetable oils, nuts, and seeds you eat.

BRAINLESS FOOD #3 FRIED FOOD AND FAST FOOD

The fact that fried food and fast food are bad for *any* part of your body should not come as a surprise. Diets high in these foods contribute significantly to poor health outcomes, so I recommend limiting them to less than once a week. If you crave a fast food burger or homemade fried chicken, consider treating it like a rare indulgence and not a dietary staple. The type of fat that you consume here—saturated and trans fats—has been directly associated with dementia risk in multiple large prospective studies of dementia and cognitive decline. In a 1993–2000 study of the Chicago Health and Aging Project, those participants whose saturated fat intake was in the top 20 percent (25 grams or more per day) had two to three times the risk of developing Alzheimer's disease over a four-year period.[45] They doubled and tripled their risk! A Burger King Whopper and medium fries would supply nearly this amount of saturated fat (21 grams). The risk was much more severe when eating trans fats. Participants who consumed 2 or more grams per day were three to five times more likely to develop Alzheimer's disease. This amount would be the equivalent of two large store-bought chocolate chip cookies.

Though we all know that fast food is bad for us, national surveys are alarming and indicate that we're eating it at an increasing rate. In 2010, the average share of the food budget spent on fast food meals and snacks was 27 percent, up from 24 percent in 1999. At the same time, the food budget spent on homemade meals and snacks declined from 25 percent to 23 percent. This closely corresponds to national food-consumption surveys, which find that 26.5 percent of adults report that they eat fast food. So who eats this the most? Numbers were highest in young adults, African Americans, households with higher incomes, those living in the suburbs, and residents of the South and Midwest.

Even more disconcerting (though perhaps not surprising) from a public health perspective is that when researchers compared the overall diets of fast food eaters to those who didn't indulge, the former were higher in total calories as well as the total and percentage of calories eaten from total fat, saturated fat, carbohydrates, and added sugars. Men ate 500 more total calories per day and women consumed 226 more. Fast food eaters were also lower in essential micronutrients such as vitamin A, carotenoids, vitamin C, magnesium, and calcium—some of which are important for brain health. Multiple prospective studies have shown that fast food contributes to increased weight gain over the adult years and to increased rates of obesity, heart disease, and diabetes. In a Harvard study of 111,631 nurses and male health professionals who were followed for twenty-five years, those who ate fried food four to six times a week had a 39 percent increased risk of diabetes and a 23 percent increased risk of coronary heart disease.[46] These increases were largely mediated through higher obesity, hypertension, and high cholesterol levels.

Since the 1960s, fried and fast foods have significantly contributed to the amount of saturated and trans fats that Americans eat—but this is no longer the case for trans fats. Since 2006, the FDA has required companies to list trans fats on nutrition labels, and consequently trans fats have been reduced in food products by 86 percent. The FDA has mandated that by 2018, trans fats be eliminated from *all* manufactured foods, which reduces concerns over the adverse health effects of trans fats. Keep in mind that although the US consumption of saturated fat has dropped from 12.2 percent of total calories in 1989 to 10.8 percent of calories in 2010, it is still higher than the 9.8 percent target set by the US Office of Disease Prevention and Health Promotion in Healthy People 2020 and the 7 percent intake level of the traditional Mediterranean diet.

BRAINLESS FOOD #4: PASTRIES AND SWEETS

If you have a sweet tooth, don't despair. There's little scientific research on how pastries and sugary foods affect our cognitive health and no direct evidence to recommend that you remove them from your diet to protect against cognitive decline and Alzheimer's disease. That said, there *are* plenty of other reasons to limit these foods to no more than five servings per week.

Pastries and sweets are full of unhealthy fats, simple carbohydrates, and salt. They are also high in calories with little nutritive value in return, and contribute to being overweight and to diets that are lower in brain-healthy foods and nutrients. Sugar and other simple carbohydrates that make up the refined grains in pastries and other sweets cause spikes in blood sugar that lead to inflammation and can damage the heart's arteries. I'm talking about candy and candy bars, sweetened beverages and sports drinks, ice cream, cookies, pies, cakes, and ready-to-eat cereals. Sweetened beverages are the largest source of added sugar in the US diet. In fact, on average, Americans consume 22 teaspoons (92 grams) of added sugar a day. To put this in perspective, the American Heart Association's current recommendations are 6 teaspoons (25 grams) per day for women and 9 teaspoons (38 grams) per day for men. In a study of 11,733 US adults who participated in the National Health and Nutrition Examination Survey (NHANES) III from 1988 to 2006, compared to participants who ate less than 10 percent of their calories from added sugar, those who consumed 25 percent or more of calories from added sugar had nearly three times the risk of death from cardiovascular diseases over 15 years.[47] The vast majority (71 percent) of these participants consumed 10 percent or more of their calories from added sugar. When grocery shopping, get into the habit of looking at the nutrition label and choosing products that have low amounts of added sugar or, as it's regularly disguised, "carbohydrate."

CAFFEINE: CAN IT HURT OR HELP YOUR MIND?

Caffeine has received heaps of attention in the field of dementia, since the stimulant directly affects the brain and central nervous system with an immediate boosting effect on the neurotransmitters acetylcholine, serotonin, adrenaline, and dopamine. These neurotransmitters are part of complex systems that involve your cognition, movement, and frame of mind. Caffeine is shown to increase alertness and mood and to decrease pain and muscle fatigue. Most dietary sources of caffeine come from coffee, tea, cola, energy drinks, and chocolate. It's added to most energy drinks (and some medications), but it occurs naturally in the leaves, seeds, and fruits of twenty-eight species of tea leaves, kola nuts, coffee beans, and cocoa beans.

A recent randomized trial of forty-three young adults, with a mean age of twenty-eight years old, nicely demonstrated caffeine's cognitive effects.[48] Subjects were given a battery of tests after consuming one cup of either caffeinated coffee (50 milligrams of caffeine) or decaffeinated coffee at two different testing sessions one week apart. Both the researchers and the participants were blinded as to what kind of beverage they were given before each testing period. The study results showed that the caffeinated coffee improved cognitive performance on tests that measured planning abilities, creative thinking, memory, and reaction times. It's safe to say, then, that a cup of coffee before a meeting or hopping in the car to drive to work may help you perform better and get to the office more safely. It could also help you focus better while making your to-do list for the day and helping your children do their homework. These are short-term effects on the brain, however, and don't necessarily extend to protecting the brain against neurodegenerative disease.

Because of these cognitive-enhancing properties, researchers have investigated caffeine as a potential drug to combat decline in cognitive function in older age. The results of animal studies provide possible biologic mechanisms to support this research. Caffeine given to rodents improved their memory function, and their brains had lower levels of amyloid plaque formation, less oxidative damage to neuronal membranes, and increased length and density of dendrites, or nerve-cell extensions, in the hippocampus.

There are no randomized trials of the effects of caffeine alone for the prevention of cognitive decline or dementia, and prospective epidemiological studies are not consistent enough to make recommendations. Some of these studies report effects only in women. The levels of caffeine needed for reported benefits vary greatly across studies—from as low as 16.5 milligrams per week to as high as 371 milligrams per day. The fact that some studies don't show any effect at 100 milligrams of caffeine per day (the equivalent of a cup of coffee) but others do raises suspicion about the validity of the findings. If caffeine truly protected the brain against neurodegenerative disease processes, then we would expect to see a consistent level of benefit across all these studies. Such inconsistencies cause concern that the observed protective relations may be due to factors related to caffeine consumption rather than the caffeine itself. For example, coffee consumption, which is the largest source of caffeine in our diets, rises dramatically from age twenty to age sixty, at which point it drops. This raises the question as to whether whatever causes some individuals to stop drinking coffee (for instance, gastrointestinal conditions, sleep disturbances, or other illnesses) may also lead to the development of dementia.

BRAINLESS FOOD #5: ADVANCED GLYCATION END PRODUCTS

Advanced glycation end products (AGEs) are pathogenic compounds in the body that form through normal metabolic processes, but they can be introduced through diet and smoking, too. The typical westernized diet—featuring a lot of processed and manufactured foods, fast foods, and high-heat cooking methods—has led to excessive consumption of AGEs in the United States and other industrialized nations. Case in point: a study of New York City residents found that the daily average consumption of AGEs was twice that of what's considered healthy (14,700 kilounits per day versus 7,340 kilounits).[49]

AGEs occur from multiple chemical reactions involving proteins, sugars, and lipids. More are formed with older age and health conditions that promote high blood sugar and oxidative stress. Researchers began taking an interest in AGEs about fifteen years ago, since they were much higher in patients with diabetes and kidney problems. High levels of AGEs cause inflammation and oxidative stress, the underlying mechanisms for most chronic diseases, including Alzheimer's disease. Several studies have found that increased levels of AGEs are associated with faster decline in cognitive abilities with older age.

The food you eat influences the levels of AGEs in your body that ultimately affect your brain. They influence normal cell function in a way that makes cells more susceptible to damage and premature aging. Animal studies have shown that dietary AGEs increase amyloid plaques in the brain regions involved in Alzheimer's disease. In both animal and human studies, restricting AGEs that come from food has effectively decreased inflammation markers and oxidative stress and lowered blood sugar levels.

AGEs occur naturally in many foods, but heat processing, especially high and/or dry heat, substantially increases the levels. Animal-derived foods that are high in fat and protein, such as meats (especially red meats), are key sources of AGEs because these compounds tend to form through the cooking process. High-temperature cooking methods that brown or char foods, such as grilling, roasting, frying, and broiling, contribute to the large amounts of AGEs that we get from our diets. Fast food is another significant source of excessive AGE levels in our diet because it's high in protein and fat and subjected to high heat when those burgers and chicken nuggets are made. Packaged and highly processed sugary foods are also high in AGEs.

The good news is that you can significantly decrease the AGEs you consume based on what you eat and how you cook. A diet that's low in AGEs is high in vegetables, legumes, fruits, and grains and low in cheese, fast and processed foods, and meats prepared primarily through boiling, sautéing, and baking (for instance, chicken baked at 350°F rather than grilled or broiled). Furthermore, marinating meat in lemon or vinegar solutions (high in pH) for an hour before cooking can cut AGEs by half. Many Mediterranean and Asian dishes are prepared using these kinds of marinades. Foods with naturally lower AGEs include bananas, apples, beans, bell peppers, mushrooms, and smoked salmon. Foods with high AGE levels include broiled hot dogs, grilled steak, thin-crust pizza, McDonald's Filet-O-Fish, and an open-face cheese melt. AGEs are just one more reason to limit fast foods, meats, sweets, and pastries. With just a little more effort, you can learn to replace them with healthier alternatives, like berries, nuts, and beans.

CHAPTER 6

Comparing the Mediterranean, DASH, and MIND Diets

As I've noted, studying dietary patterns in relationship to disease — and then turning those research-based findings into a diet that helps patients in real life and real time — is a relatively new area of public health research. In fact, scientific investigations that have done this to any extent have focused mostly on the Mediterranean diet and the DASH diet. While both the Mediterranean and DASH diets have been shown to improve heart health, and while we know that a healthy heart lends to a healthy mind, these diets aren't specific to the literature on nutrition and the brain.

To address this gap, my colleagues and I at Rush and Harvard Universities developed a new diet called the MIND (Mediterranean-DASH Intervention for Neurodegenerative Delay) diet. The MIND diet incorporates many of the basic components of the Mediterranean and DASH diets but with modifications that reflect the best scientific evidence on nutrition and the prevention of dementia — information that you currently hold in your hands. And because the Mediterranean and DASH diets have influenced the MIND diet, I wanted to take this time to explain all three so that you can see how each informs the others.

In this chapter, you'll learn about the extent to which the foods we've discussed (and that you'll prepare in part II) will help ward off debilitating cognitive decline and dementia. The effectiveness of the DASH and Mediterranean diets for protection against cardiovascular-related diseases has been established in study after study—including in randomized clinical trials, the most rigorous type of study design. But because the MIND diet is relatively new, our large randomized trials are still underway. By following the advice in this book, you are truly on the cutting edge of brain health.

WHERE IT ALL BEGAN: THE MEDITERRANEAN DIET

The Mediterranean diet is significant to heart and brain health not only because of its demonstrated ability to cut disease rates, but because it has changed how researchers study the relationship between diet and brain. It's now one of the most clinically cited diets for a strong heart as well as for overall health. It has had a significant influence on the MIND diet, too.

The first person to link the Mediterranean diet to health was an American scientist named Ancel Keys in the 1950s. He initiated the Seven Countries Study, an international study aimed at investigating the effects of diet and culture on coronary heart disease.[50] Over a thirty-year period, the study followed 12,763 men age forty to fifty-nine years old from sixteen different regions: two regions in Greece, three in Italy, five in the former Yugoslavia, two in Japan, two in Finland, one in the Netherlands, and one in the United States. To the surprise of Keys and many other researchers, the study found that coronary heart disease rates were much lower in Greece and Italy than even in the wealthy New York City population, despite disparities in economic development and healthcare. In fact, up until recently, Greece had one of the lowest mortality rates in the world, particularly as compared to Spain, the United Kingdom, and the United States. This was largely due to lower rates of coronary heart disease and many cancers, including breast, prostate, ovarian, and colon cancer. (The reason Greece's mortality rate is no longer quite so low may be attributable to the westernization of the diet.)

Of course, there are many cultural practices that are different between the traditional Mediterranean populations and the westernized world, including more daily physical activity, a lower-stress lifestyle, and stronger community ties. But the Seven Countries Study identified diet as a primary factor in the Mediterranean countries' lower disease rates. The traditional Mediterranean diet has a high amount of fat; depending on the country, the range is 30 to 40 percent of total energy intake, and it is mostly olive oil, which is high in monounsaturated fat. The amount of saturated fat in the Mediterranean diet is low, less than 7 percent of total calories. This compares to the US Department of Agriculture recommendation of 30 percent of calories from total fat and 9 percent from saturated fat. To give some perspective, for a person who consumes 2,000 calories per day, a single Burger King Whopper with cheese would provide 74 percent of the US recommended total fat intake and 92 percent of the saturated fat intake. A grilled 5-ounce T-bone steak would yield about half of the recommended intake of these fats (42 percent of total, 55 percent of saturated).

The best scientific evidence has since verified that the Mediterranean countries' traditional diets accounted for their comparably low rates of death. In fact, a Harvard study of 6,137 female and 11,278 male health professionals with cardiovascular disease found that those who most closely followed the Mediterranean diet (the top 20 percent of Mediterranean diet scores) had a 19 percent lower risk of death from any cause compared with those who followed the diet the least (bottom 20 percent of scores).[51] They also had a 15 percent lower risk of death from cardiovascular and cancer causes, and among women specifically, the risk of death from all other causes combined was lower by 21 percent. Included among the other causes of death were chronic obstructive pulmonary disease, diabetes, Alzheimer's disease, Parkinson's disease, pneumonia, cirrhosis, and other chronic liver diseases.

The Harvard study is an observational cohort study, and as I've discussed earlier, this type of study can never fully eliminate all the factors that are associated with diet that may contribute to the lower death rate. The PREDIMED trial of the Mediterranean diet, however, provides even stronger evidence of its favorable health effects because the 7,447 study participants, all at high cardiovascular risk, were randomly assigned to a diet: the Mediterranean diet supplemented with olive oil, the Mediterranean diet supplemented with nuts, or a low-fat control diet. The random assignment effectively eliminated the contribution of other healthy lifestyle behaviors to health outcomes. By this I mean that, for example, exercisers were randomly assigned to all three diets so that exercise and diet were completely unrelated.

The results of the PREDIMED trial were so successful that the trial was stopped early, in 2010, after an average of 4.8 years of follow-up. Compared to the low-fat diet group, the Mediterranean diet group that supplemented with olive oil experienced a 30 percent reduction in the occurrence of major cardiovascular events (myocardial infarction, stroke, and death from cardiovascular causes), and the Mediterranean diet group that supplemented with nuts had a 28 percent reduction in cardiovascular events. The magnitude of this effect is similar to the risk reduction obtained with statin drugs. Further studies of the PREDIMED trial found that the Mediterranean diet groups had significant reductions compared to the low-fat group in blood pressure, inflammation, obesity, and waist circumference, and a 28 percent reduction in the development of diabetes. And best of all, no adverse effects of the diet were reported (the use of statin drugs, on the other hand, has been reported to increase the occurrence of diabetes). This just goes to show how important adopting a healthy diet is to optimum health. Regardless of whether you are on statins or other medications, eating a diet that's plant-based and low in saturated fats and sweets can make a huge difference in how you maintain your health throughout your life.

For our purposes, the Mediterranean diet was also one of the first dietary patterns investigated in relation to dementia. In 2006, Nikolaos Scarmeas, a neurologist at Columbia University who's a native of Greece, reported on a study that examined the dietary habits of a Manhattan population that initially didn't have dementia and followed them for an average of four years for development of Alzheimer's disease.[52] The study population was largely of black and Hispanic ethnicity, and not of Mediterranean origin. Consumption of olive oil, a primary characteristic of the Mediterranean diet, was almost nonexistent in this study population. Nevertheless, when the participants' diets were scored according to the Mediterranean dietary pattern, those with the highest scores had the lowest risk of developing Alzheimer's disease. Later studies by Scarmeas's scientific team found that higher adherence to the Mediterranean diet in this population was associated with reduced risks of mild cognitive impairment and stroke. What's more, images of the brain in a smaller group from the population showed less atrophy. Other studies around the world, including my own Chicago studies of diet and dementia in the Memory and Aging Project and Chicago Health and Aging Project cohorts, reported positive results, too. The findings of the PREDIMED study and these large prospective studies yield strong evidence that the Mediterranean diet pattern can prevent dementia.

More than twenty countries surround the Mediterranean basin, a region noted for olive-growing and wine-making. And while specifics in Mediterranean diets vary, they have the same basic components:

High consumption of olive oil, vegetables, fruits, legumes, and whole grains

Moderate consumption of alcohol and dairy products, mostly in the form of wine, feta cheese, and yogurt

Low consumption of sweets, meat (especially red meat), and meat products

Moderate consumption of seafood (varying in type throughout the region by availability), with higher consumption in the coastal populations

Rare consumption of butter, margarine, shortening, or vegetable oils other than olive oil

Whole-grain bread at every meal

Local produce in season

Primarily sautéing and stir-frying as cooking methods

Minimally processed, seasonal, and locally grown foods, which help maximize the fiber, nutrients, and bioactive compounds obtained from the diet

FOR HEART HEALTH AND MORE:
THE DASH DIET

Another major diet shown to improve health is the DASH (Dietary Approaches to Stop Hypertension) diet. The DASH diet was developed in the mid-1990s by US scientists to lower blood pressure and has been tested in multiple randomized clinical trials sponsored by the National Institutes of Health (NIH). The immensely successful results of the diet for preventing hypertension and diabetes, as well as for weight loss and reduced markers of inflammation and oxidative stress, have resulted in its endorsement by the American Heart Association as well as the NIH National Heart, Lung, and Blood Institute. For the last six years, *U.S. News & World Report* has ranked DASH the number one healthiest diet.

Results of the first DASH diet trial were published in 1997.[53] Researchers enrolled 459 adults with blood pressures in the prehypertensive or hypertensive range in the trial. Participants were randomized to receive prepared meals for one of three different diets: (1) a control diet that was low in fruits, vegetables, and dairy products, and with a fat content that was typical of the average American diet (total fat, 37 percent of calories; saturated fat, 16 percent of calories), (2) a diet rich in fruits and vegetables, or (3) the DASH diet, which was rich in fruits and vegetables but also had reduced saturated and total fat, including low-fat dairy products.

The trial's results were amazing. After eight weeks, among the participants who had blood pressures in the hypertensive range (greater than 140 mmHg systolic or greater than 90 mmHg diastolic blood pressure levels), the DASH diet resulted in reductions of 11.4 mmHg systolic and 5.5 mmHg diastolic blood pressure compared with that of controls. Over all the participants, hypertensive and prehypertensive, the DASH diet significantly reduced systolic and diastolic blood pressure over that in controls by 5.5 and 3.0 mmHg, respectively. The fruits and vegetables diet also resulted in significant blood pressure reductions, but the reductions were much smaller than those in the DASH diet group. In a later blood pressure trial investigating the effects of sodium reductions alone or in combination with the DASH diet, both the DASH diet and dietary sodium restriction to 100 mg per day were effective in bringing about large decreases in blood pressure, but the greatest effect was when the two dietary measures were combined.

Just as in the PREDIMED study, the DASH diet has also been shown to benefit cognitive function in a randomized trial called ENCORE (Exercise and Nutritional Interventions for Cardiovascular Health).[54] This trial, designed to study the diet's effects on cardiovascular outcomes in hypertensive and obese subjects, administered cognitive tests to a subset of 124 participants at the outset and again after four months. Some of the participants were randomized to follow the DASH diet, some to DASH plus weight management (including exercise and calorie reduction), some to weight management alone, and others to the usual-diet control group. After just four months on the intervention, those participants on the DASH diet performed better on tests of cognitive speed than the control group. Even more striking, the group that received both the DASH diet and weight management interventions exhibited superior performance on tests of memory and problem solving, and the effects were particularly strong among those who also increased their aerobic fitness and lost the most weight.

The development of the DASH diet was based on years of scientific studies that observed lower blood pressure levels in vegetarians, as well as among individuals who consumed diets that had these characteristics:

Lower in fats (particularly saturated fats), red meat, sweets, and sugar-containing beverages

Moderate in alcohol

Higher in dietary intake of fiber and minerals such as magnesium, potassium, and calcium

Emphasized fruits, vegetables, and low-fat dairy foods

Included whole grains, poultry, fish, and nuts

Sodium is a key factor known to increase blood pressure, but the original DASH diet did not include reduced sodium.

THE BEST OF ALL WORLDS: THE MIND DIET

The DASH and Mediterranean diets have demonstrated many cardiovascular and other health benefits, but neither is specific to the foods and nutrients that have been identified as playing a role in the prevention of neurodegenerative diseases like Alzheimer's disease. After all, the Mediterranean diet is a cultural diet, specific to the region, and the DASH diet was developed to prevent hypertension based on the scientific literature of nutrition and blood pressure. But what about preserving the brain?

To address the absence of a diet designed specifically for the brain, the MIND diet was created by me and my Rush colleagues, along with Dr. Frank Sacks, who was one of the originators of the DASH diet and a former mentor at the Harvard School of Public Health. MIND is an acronym for "Mediterranean-DASH Intervention for Neurodegenerative Delay." The diet includes many of the basic dietary components of the DASH and Mediterranean diets: it is plant-based, low in red meat and sweets, and low in saturated fats. As such, it is likely to reduce weight, decrease oxidative stress and inflammation, and protect the cardiovascular system, although these benefits haven't been tested as yet.

But the diet also includes modifications to the Mediterranean and DASH diets that reflect nutrients, foods, and servings related to brain health, just as I have described in this book. For example, both the Mediterranean and DASH diets include four or more servings of vegetables and three or more servings of fruit, with no distinction of type of vegetable and fruit. One key difference of the MIND diet is the recommendation of two or more vegetables per day, one of which is a leafy green vegetable. Likewise, as compared with three or more daily servings of any fruit in the DASH and Mediterranean diets, the MIND diet specifies berries. Another healthy food component of the MIND diet is the consumption of seafood at least once per week, as described in chapter 4. This compares to six or more servings per week in the Mediterranean diet. The DASH diet emphasizes dairy, which is not specified in the MIND diet.

In all, the MIND diet has fifteen dietary components: ten healthy foods to include in the diet and five unhealthy foods that should be restricted but not necessarily eliminated:

10 Healthy Foods

6+ servings per week of leafy green vegetables

1+ serving per day of other vegetables

3 servings per day of whole grains

2+ servings per week of berries

5+ servings per week of nuts

1+ serving per week of seafood

2+ servings per week of poultry

4+ servings per week of beans and legumes

Olive oil as the primary oil used

1 glass per day of wine

5 Unhealthy Foods

<5 servings per week of sweets and pastries

<4 servings per week of red meats and red-meat products

<1 serving per week of fried/fast foods

<1 serving per week of whole-fat cheese

<1 pat per day of butter or trans-fat margarine

The first reports on the MIND diet came out in 2015.[55] We used the comprehensive dietary assessments that were completed by participants of the Memory and Aging Project (MAP) to assign scores based on how closely the participants' diets followed the recommendations specified in the MIND diet. Possible scores ranged from 15 (highest adherence) to 0 (lowest adherence), although the highest score obtained in the MAP study was just over 12. Our study was based on 923 MAP participants who were unaffected by dementia at the start of the study and who also provided dietary data so that we could assign a MIND diet score. The participants ranged in age from fifty-eight to ninety-eight years old and were followed for an average of almost five years. Those participants in the top third of the MIND diet scores (8.5 to 12.5) had a 53 percent lower risk of developing Alzheimer's disease compared with those with the lowest MIND scores (2.5 to 6.5). What was also astounding was that even those with MIND scores in the intermediate range (scores of 7 and 8) had a 35 percent lower risk of Alzheimer's disease.

In the second report from the MAP study, we investigated whether the MIND diet score was associated with changes in cognitive abilities for up to ten years.[56] In analyses that controlled for other factors that could account for cognitive decline, like education, age, and physical activities, we found that *the higher the MIND diet score, the better the participants performed over time on all the cognitive tests.* Those participants who ranked in the top third of scores had a rate of cognitive decline that was equivalent to being 7.5 years younger in age!

In further analyses of the MAP study cohort, we examined whether the MIND diet was superior to the Mediterranean and DASH diets when it came to neuroprotection. We re-analyzed participants' dietary assessments to calculate scores for how closely each MAP participant followed the DASH and Mediterranean diets. We then related these scores to our measures of cognitive decline and the development of Alzheimer's disease. Both the Mediterranean and DASH diets were associated with slower decline and a lower risk of Alzheimer's disease — however, the MIND diet was more protective than either the Mediterranean or DASH diets. In fact, the protective association of the MIND diet score with cognitive decline was almost *twice as strong* as either the Mediterranean or DASH diet. The risk of Alzheimer's disease was equally reduced by about 50 percent with high scores on the MIND and Mediterranean diets, but even moderate scores on the MIND diet were significantly associated with a 35 percent reduction in the risk of developing the disease.

The findings, while exciting, need more extensive research to verify that the MIND diet protects the brain against neurodegenerative processes that cause dementia. In April 2016, we received funding from the National Institute on Aging to do just that. The grant is allowing us to test the effects of the MIND diet on cognitive decline and structural changes in the brain in a large randomized trial. A total of six hundred Boston and Chicago residents age sixty-five to eighty-four years old will be randomly assigned to one of two diet groups for a period of three years: the MIND diet plus mild calorie reduction (250 calories per day) or the typical US diet plus mild calorie reduction. This is one of the first such trials to directly test the effects of diet on cognitive aging. The results of the MIND trial should be out in 2021, when all six hundred participants have concluded the three-year intervention and we have completed the analyses. The trial results will form public health policy and dietary recommendations for healthy cognitive aging.

PART II

MIND-HEALTHY LIFESTYLE AND RECIPES

CHAPTER 7

Create Your Healthiest Life

Now that you understand the latest science on what it takes to support and preserve your brain, it's time to combine that with a simple lifestyle plan and delicious recipes to help you live your healthiest life.

In earlier chapters of the book, I laid the groundwork for what would be involved in creating a *mind-healthy* lifestyle. It's not just about what you eat, but also about making sure you exercise, get sufficient sleep, manage stress, and fill your life with relationships that support your mind, body, and goals. It's about finding the best practices for you to be at your healthiest as well as the best coping mechanisms to keep you from veering too far off track.

A healthy mind also requires a life in balance. One of the most consistent scientific findings about healthful aging in all areas — whether you're talking cardiovascular health, weight control, brain health, or bone and joint wellness — is that having a balanced lifestyle is key. There's a reason that the significant studies in this book point to a balanced dietary intake and not an extreme one. There are few foods we consider "bad," just ones that you should limit. There is no superfood or do-or-die approach here, just food groups that, when they're eaten daily or every few days, significantly decrease your chances of experiencing cognitive decline and dementia. If you think about it, it's a rather modest effort for a big payout! But that's what I suspect nature intended. Our bodies weren't designed to thrive in an environment of extremes—indulgent foods versus extreme restriction, or excessive movement versus long stretches of inactivity. There are so many ways to bring a balanced approach to enhancing your health and your mind. If you make the most of the advice and recipes in part II, you'll be off to a great start.

My goal throughout this book has been to arm you with the very best science about brain-enriching foods so that you can make smart choices to prevent cognitive decline and dementias like Alzheimer's disease—and now, it's time to round out the rest of the story. I'll turn it over to my daughter Laura, a certified personal trainer and nutrition consultant, who will help you pull all the pieces together to maintain a healthy mind and body. In this chapter, she'll outline healthy lifestyle tips that support the science from part I. These tips boil down to just five factors: weight, exercise, diet, sleep, and mindset. Doing well in just one of these areas—say, diet—will not help as much as if you do your best in all the areas. But again, balance is key. So if you can't get to the gym one afternoon, but you ate sensibly, slept well, and kept your stress under control, that's still terrific, and we want you to celebrate that, too.

The most important factor to living a mind-healthy life, however, is *you*. From here on out, your success relies on your ability to make changes, stick with them, and hold yourself responsible for your progress. Ultimately, it's not your doctor's job, or your spouse's, or your trainer's to help you avoid chronic illnesses and a poor aging process. It's yours! Every one of us faces challenges that make our days bumpier than we'd like—bad knees, family problems, issues with children, budget struggles—but you can't let them get in the way of your desire or ability to give you and your brain the best shot at a vibrant life.

WEIGHT: KNOW YOUR BMI

Not many of us enjoy talking about our weight, but for your health's sake, it is a critical conversation. How much you weigh conveys so much about how healthy you—and your mind—are. Maintaining a healthy weight lowers your risk of heart disease, diabetes, stroke, high blood pressure, and many cancers. It will also help you preserve your brain functioning. Some studies have shown that those who gain more than ten pounds after age twenty are three times more likely to develop heart disease, high blood pressure, diabetes, and gallstones than those who gain five pounds or fewer! The first step toward keeping yourself in good shape is to figure out your body mass index (BMI). A healthy BMI for both men and women is between 18 and 24. If your BMI is below 18, you are considered underweight; if it is 25 to 29 you are considered overweight; 30 to 35 is considered obese level 1; 35 to 40 is obese level 2; and 40 or higher is considered morbidly obese. Here is the formula to calculate your BMI:

(703 × weight in pounds) ÷ (height in inches × height in inches)

So a 150-pound person who is 5 feet 9 inches (69 inches) tall would calculate BMI as follows: (703 × 150) ÷ (69 × 69) = 22. Talk to your doctor if you have a BMI below 18 or above 25 to make sure there are no health conditions outside of lifestyle practices that are causing weight loss or gain. Following the guidelines for diet and exercise provided in this book will help guide you to a healthier BMI.

EXERCISE: GET MOVING

It is extremely important to find an exercise routine that you enjoy and can sustain. Exercise not only keeps your brain at peak performance but can also lower your risk of cardiovascular disease, high blood pressure and cholesterol levels, type 2 diabetes, and some cancers. Physical activity strengthens your bones and muscles and improves your overall mood, too. The American Heart Association (AHA) recommends that you get at least 150 minutes per week of moderate-intensity aerobic activity (30 minutes on five days of the week), or 75 minutes a week at a vigorous activity (25 minutes on three days of the week). What is the difference between moderate and vigorous activity? Everyone's fitness level is different, but in general, if you are still able to carry on a conversation while you exercise, as you could on a brisk walk, this would be considered moderate-intensity exercise. However, if you are unable to say more than a few words because of breathlessness, as you would in a spin class, your exercise level has moved into the vigorous range.

It is important that you get aerobic exercise through the activities you love — biking, dancing, hiking, playing basketball, walking — and do them often. Make it the best part of your day. Humans are designed and built to move, and exercise is one of the most important things that you can do for yourself.

Beyond aerobic exercise, the AHA also recommends resistance training at least twice a week. Resistance training is great for strengthening your muscles and bones and improving your mood and self-esteem. In older adults it has been shown to increase walking speed and to prevent falls and the need for assistance with basic activities of daily living. There is even some evidence that it may help prevent cognitive decline. Resistance training also protects against type 2 diabetes by decreasing the amount of fat around your organs, and it may enhance your cardiovascular health by reducing resting blood pressure and improving blood cholesterol levels.

If you're new to resistance training (or intimidated by it), find a qualified fitness professional at your local gym or community center to help you get started. Resistance training is ideally performed two to four times a week, spaced with a day or two in between workouts. Your muscle tissue breaks down after a muscle-building session, and it needs this time of rest to repair. Aim to hit all muscle groups at least once a week. Just be sure to have a balanced meal or snack of carbs and protein no more than 45 minutes after your workout to help your muscles rebuild and recover with reduced soreness. Some examples of a good post-workout snack are a protein shake with fruit, an apple with peanut butter, or whole-grain crackers with hummus and two hard-boiled eggs.

Understand Your Brain-Body Principles

There are many commonalities between what it takes to maintain a healthy brain and what it takes to maintain a strong and resilient body. If you can keep the following six fitness principles in mind while creating your exercise plan, you'll be able to do both.

1. *Principle of individual variance.* Everyone's body is built differently. Whether because of gender, genetics, age, or past experiences, what works for one person may be different from what works for another. Just as some people are visual learners while others benefit from verbal learning, various individual factors contribute to how we excel. Pay attention to your body's strengths and weaknesses, and make an exercise plan based on your needs and abilities. For example, if you have bad knees and a high body weight, running may not be the best exercise for you, but weight training and Pilates could help improve your knee pain and keep you strong and fit.

2. *Principle of overload.* When you aim to challenge your brain so it will learn and develop, you must expose it to a certain

level of new information. The same goes for your body and muscles. To see increased muscle or cardiovascular strength, you need a certain amount of stress or overload. This means that your muscles must work for a longer period of time or at a higher intensity level than they're used to—as when your muscles burn from doing repetitions with weights or your heart rate is higher than is comfortable. This can be done by adding a few more reps than you have been performing, or increasing the weight you are lifting by a couple of pounds. There is no better feeling than when your mind starts to doubt your capabilities and your body pushes through. This is when change and growth happen; just be sure that this overload is gradual and consistent.

3. *Principle of progression.* Have you ever studied so hard for an exam that your brain just turned to mush and you could not take in any more information? The same thing happens to your muscles. If you work out too hard, and for too long, your body will face adverse effects like injury or muscle damage—and, most likely, full-body fatigue. Similarly, if you do not overload your muscles enough—for example, if you hit the gym only once a week—you will not reap the benefits of what you are trying to accomplish. The best way to see healthy gains is by gradually and consistently overloading and pushing your muscles and body.

4. *Principle of adaptation.* When we first learn math, we start with simple addition. After a few weeks we learn to subtract, then we learn to multiply and divide, and so on until we are learning complex calculus and algebra. The brain adapts and becomes more capable the more we challenge it. The same goes for your muscles and cardiovascular system. If you run five miles every

day at the same pace on the same trail and never change your routine, running that five miles will become easy and your body will adapt. Other areas of your body may become weak and underperform, too. Our bodies and minds need variation to keep adapting and getting stronger. When you have been performing the same exercise routine for four to six weeks, such as running five miles at the same pace, your body will no longer be challenged the way you were when you first started running. After four to six weeks, vary your run by adding ten interval sprints at the end of the run, increasing the distance by a mile or two, or choosing a steeper trail to run on. When we adapt and become physically stronger, it opens up our minds and bodies to become stronger and more efficient.

5. *Principal of "use it or lose it."* If you don't practice a foreign language, you will not get better—in fact, you may lose those language skills over time if they are neglected. Same goes for exercise. If you do not work your muscles, they atrophy. Stay on top of movement and resistance training, or your body (and brain!) will lose all the effects of the hard work you've done.

6. *The principle of specificity.* If you want to become better at sudoku, you should regularly practice sudoku. In this way, your mind will quickly learn the methods and patterns needed to master that specific skill. Similarly, if you want to become better at shooting basketball free throws, you'll need to frequently practice shooting free throws. Whatever your exercise focus, practice it and learn everything you can about it. Consult a trainer if possible, but fitness partners can also make excellent coaches. Having someone support and guide you to help focus on what you want is the best way to meet your plans for a healthy mind and body.

WORKOUT AND MOTIVATION TIPS

It can be tough to squeeze in exercise time. Here are some tips to help make it a bit easier.

- *Buy proper workout shoes and clothes.* Wearing appropriate attire can help prevent injuries and regulate your body temperature. In addition, dressing for success puts your mind in the right place to give it your all.

- *Find a partner or workout environment you love.* Fitness trainers, group classes, and workout buddies go a long way toward motivating you and holding you accountable. Gyms, workout centers, clubs—they all have their own welcoming communities that can become places of support for all areas of your life.

- *Consider your fitness needs at the moment.* What do you want from your exercise? Weight loss? Strength? Rehabilitation of an injury? Stress reduction? Mind stimulation? And how much time are you willing to commit to this? Decide what your physical needs are at this moment in your life, and then find the classes, activities, or trainer to help you meet them.

- *Identify your obstacles.* Be realistic about what you can achieve, and set yourself up for success. Figure out how you'll deal with known obstacles before they get in the way. For instance, if you have a demanding work schedule, commit to an hour twice a week, and make it during a time period when it can't be canceled, no matter how your day is scheduled. If you have an injury or chronic issue, like back pain, see a trainer with experience in this to help you overcome it.

- *Give yourself a focus.* Set goals, big or small, to work toward. Aim for an activity with a set end point, like running a race, performing an hour-long exercise, or doing a particular number of push-ups. Once you reach that point, set another goal, and reward yourself with a treat like a massage or new workout outfit.

- *Keep a calendar.* People tend to think that they work out more than they actually do. Keep a calendar of your daily workouts to remind you how hard you're working and to determine whether there's a pattern to when you're not that into it. This will help push you when you need it as well as show you just how far you've come.

- *Accept change.* Change is one of the hardest challenges to face. It disrupts everything in you and can be scary. The exciting thing about the world of fitness is the constant challenge to physically improve. It opens you up and allows you to move forward with new confidence.

DIET: CREATE MEAL PLANS THAT WORK FOR YOU

Though this book outlines very specific foods to prevent cognitive decline and dementia, you'll need to know a few dietary basics beyond those in part I so that you can flesh out your meal plans each week. In addition to preparing the delicious recipes provided in this book, it's important to make sure your meals are nutritious when you are eating out. If your plate is made up of foods that come straight from the ground or a tree (after being cleaned, of course), you are eating meals that will help fight disease. Other foods, such as pasta, cheese, and bread, have beneficial nutrients as well, but they have undergone processing, so be aware of undesirable added ingredients such as salt, sugar, and preservatives. Try to limit your intake of these foods throughout the day. For example, a turkey sandwich is often viewed as a "healthy" meal. But the bread and even the turkey might be highly processed, and the sandwich might contain only a half serving of vegetables (lettuce and tomato). A better option would be a grilled chicken breast with a quinoa-vegetable salad.

A diet that is nourishing for your brain and overall health contains the following components:

Foods that are mostly made at home

Foods that contain no added sugars, including high-fructose corn syrup

A variety of fruits and vegetables every day

A variety of healthy fats from foods like avocados, nuts, fish, and vegetable oils (especially olive oil)

Minimal processed foods, including cookies, chips, and fast foods

Plan Ahead

When it comes to eating well, exercising, and living a healthy life, planning is essential. Maintaining a good diet is nearly impossible without some basic meal planning: creating a menu, making a grocery list, and prepping meals ahead of time. Studies show that healthy eaters are consistent in the foods they eat and the dishes they create. They may eat oatmeal and berries every morning for breakfast, a spinach salad and soup every day for lunch, and protein and veggies for dinner—with slight variations. Though our bodies need variety to truly thrive, the larger point is that predictability in the timing and composition of your diet helps your body know what to expect and when, and this helps regulate your metabolism, as well as other body systems. This highlights a major upside of turning your diet into a regimented discipline: it will help you maintain a healthy weight as well as keep your body and mind running efficiently.

We strongly suggest that you get into the routine of meal planning. By making it a habit, in time you will find it to be second nature. Here are some tips to make it easy:

- *Plan your menu for the week.* Set aside time at the beginning of each week to write out a weekly menu, including what you'll eat if you go out for dinner or dig into leftovers. Leave as little opportunity for a last-minute scramble as you can. Write out a grocery list for all meal ingredients.

- *Prepare.* Take a few hours after you do your weekly shopping to prep, chop, and even cook large portions so that you don't have to fuss when you're busier.

- *Consider a grocery-store delivery service.* A service like this can be invaluable if you're pressed for time or on a budget, because you will not be tempted to grab unnecessary "impulse" items that rack up the bill.

- *Read labels.* Reading labels doesn't help you understand the best nutrients; it helps you weed out the bad ones. Avoid buying products with unnecessary or even harmful ingredients. If you're buying maple syrup, for example, make sure it's pure. No pure maple syrup label will list caramel color, glucose, and high-fructose corn syrup.

- *Be aware of, and diversify, your daily intake.* If you eat an egg sandwich for breakfast, try not to eat a sandwich for lunch or dinner. Look to other sources of carbohydrates and proteins, such as legumes, brown rice, or quinoa. If you're invited to a pizza party for dinner, eat a light breakfast, then fruit and vegetables at lunch so that you fill up on healthy food ahead of time.

- *Let yourself feel hungry.* Don't let yourself *stay* hungry, but do train your eating habits so that your body uses food efficiently and triggers hunger when you need more fuel. This means not overeating at meals and getting a balanced mix of carbohydrates, fats, and protein at most meals and snack times.

- *Avoid temptation.* If it helps to remove yourself from situations that require too much willpower, do it. If it means setting aside your plate when you feel full and storing the leftovers, do that, too. Go for walks or find activities to distract you if you tend to eat when you're not hungry. Do not bring foods into your home that will trigger you to overeat, and never snack out of a box or bag—always portion it out.

- *Be prepared for snack attacks.* Carry nuts, fruit, vegetables, and trail mix with you so you can eat nutritious food when you need it. Pack a lunch if you're traveling to an area with only fast food spots, and choose restaurants with healthy menus so that you can satisfy your cravings and dietary needs. When you are going to a restaurant, look at the menu ahead of time and pick out a nutritious light meal so that you're not tempted by unhealthy options.

- *Get into the mindset of being a person who eats well.* Know your weaknesses, and don't focus on how hard it is to change. Think about how much healthier your brain and body will be.

Become Someone Who Cooks

Yes, there will be times when you don't feel like cooking, reheating, or even assembling prepared meals, and that's okay. But there *are* ways to get yourself in the mood, even on your laziest or busiest days.

The most important thing is to get comfortable in the kitchen. Don't let meal prep intimidate you. This is your domain now. You've got this. If you're confident in this space, and particularly with a knife, you'll feel more motivated to chop, dice, and slice on a daily basis. In fact, most cooks will tell you that they find it relaxing to cut up food—almost therapeutic. Buy yourself a decent chef's knife, learn proper cutting techniques (there are lots of simple tutorials on YouTube), and then practice every day. You may find that cooking becomes the most relaxing part of your day.

Food is much tastier, more nutritious, and easier to cook when it's in season, so try to buy seasonal—and local, too, if you can, to support your regional farmers. Pay attention to what's in your fridge. You want to feel inspired when you open the refrigerator, so keep it as neat and clutter-free as you can. Throw away old food that's not only bad to eat but discouraging to look at. Keep track of what you have stocked in your pantry; spices, dried herbs, and canned goods can be quickly made into a tasty last-minute meal.

Get your family involved! It can be frustrating to work hard on a meal only to watch your kids or spouse turn up their noses once it's served. So when you create your weekly dinner plan, ask everyone in the house for ideas. Even better, ask them to help you in the kitchen to boost enthusiasm.

Being present and mindful makes the experience of cooking rewarding and enjoyable. Taste, smell, and listen to the food as you prepare it. This is the best way to understand and appreciate not just what you're eating but how cooking works. Tasting your food throughout the process helps you recognize the different stages of cooking and how to season a dish just so. Smelling your food is important to understanding doneness, stage of ripeness, and seasoning. Listening to the sounds of your vegetables sautéing, steaming, and roasting gives you an idea of how close they are to being done. If you make it a point to value the cooking process, you'll learn more about your food than you thought possible.

Finally, remember that cooking is a great, generous, loving gesture. Connecting over delicious, high-quality food that keeps everyone happy and healthy is one of the best gifts you can give to your loved ones.

Healthy Environments Feed Healthy Habits

Your behavior toward food, exercise, relationships, and stress is formed at a very early age. From the first nibbles you devoured as a baby to the foods you enjoyed at family gatherings growing up, how and what you eat have been influenced by other people's preferences and habits. So, if you came from a household with health-conscious parents who made nourishing meals, provided nuts, fruit, and vegetables as snacks, and generally encouraged a positive relationship with food, you are more likely to have the same approach as an adult. If you grew up learning that fast food and frozen meals were the norm, snacks came from a box, and meal-time happened in front of the TV, then those are most likely your habits as an adult.

If your upbringing was more like the latter example, fear not—you are not doomed! Your habits can be changed for the better, and you have the power to make sure your current environment supports brain-healthy eating. Take the initiative and create a community, at work and at home, that positively influences your lifestyle. Limit social temptations that keep you from the gym and surround you with junk food at home, work, and social events. Most loved ones want what is best for you, but if your inner circle doesn't get it, set some ground rules. Give them specific tips so they can help you. Ask them to cheer on the positive changes you are making. A big misconception is that fit, healthy, and mentally sharp people are born that way and that it's easy for them to maintain their healthy habits. But that's not true. Nobody has superhuman willpower or strength to help them stay disciplined. Rather, these people live within an environment that fosters health. Practice good eating habits through consistent meal timing and meal com-position. Get in the habit of exercising regularly and getting ade-quate sleep. Most important, be mindful and implement positive coping mechanisms to stress. Who knows? Maybe once your loved ones see all the progress you have made, they will be inspired to join in!

WORK IT OUT

If you are an average American adult, you spend about a third of your life at work, so your work environment plays a big role in your physical health. Think about what you are snacking on for a third of your life when there's a regular rotation of sweets and pastries on the conference table. How active are you if you sit at a desk all day and, rather than going to the gym after work, you go out for drinks with coworkers? If your office life is inhibiting your healthy lifestyle behaviors, focus on what you can do to change the problem and keep yourself on track. Here are some tips:

- Restrict sweets, pastries, and candy to once a month in the office; anything else can be donated.

- Bring in healthy snacks, such as vegetables and hummus or fruit and nuts.

- Set an alarm to go off every hour to remind yourself to get up and move around.

- Ask your company to cover employees' yoga, spin, or exercise classes at a local gym.

- Lead "walking meetings" instead of sitting in a conference room or restaurant.

- Start workplace fitness challenges like number of stairs climbed, or a softball team or running group. If you don't know where to begin, you can recruit local fitness professionals for advice, guidance, and/or training.

SLEEP: PRIORITIZE YOUR ZZZ'S

It may seem obvious, but we all need quality sleep to rest and restore our bodies and brains. Sleep plays a critical role in immune health, memory, metabolism, learning, and other vital functions. Lack of sleep can lead to a host of health problems, including obesity and early mortality. The National Heart, Lung, and Blood Institute recommends that adults, including the elderly, get seven to eight hours of sleep a night.

There are many things you can do to maximize your best sleep efforts and achieve good sleep hygiene. Follow these simple steps to get the rest your body needs so that you can mentally and physically thrive:

- *Avoid caffeine, alcohol, and other stimulants that may interrupt sleep.* You should have no caffeine four to six hours before bedtime. Limit alcoholic beverages to no more than one or two per day and avoid consumption within three hours before bedtime.

- *Establish a bedtime routine that helps tell your body to sleep.* This can include light stretches, a hot bath or shower, or reading.

- *Make your bedroom ideal for sound sleep.* Invest in blackout curtains, a comfortable mattress, and pillows. The temperature should be cool and comfortable, and the air well ventilated. Reserve the bed for sleeping and sex only. Try not to bring electronics and work materials to bed, especially computers, tablets, and smartphones with bright lights.

- *Keep your internal clock regular.* Going to bed and waking up at the same time each day is the best way to set your internal clock. Set your alarm clock to a consistent time, even on weekends.

- *Exercise no later than three hours before bedtime, if possible.* Eat light meals in the evening and stay well hydrated throughout the day for peaceful sleep.

MINDSET: MAKE HAPPINESS A CHOICE

A healthy mind is a happy mind, and a big part of maintaining a blissful state as you age is learning how to respond to stress, anxiety, and life challenges in a positive way. When you're faced with a problem, it's going to shape you in some way. You can let it either strengthen your resilience or pull you down a path of physical and emotional sabotage (think binge eating, binge drinking, social isolation, making excuses, overworking, being sedentary). Like it or not, stress affects your diet, mood, exercise regimen, relationships, and sleep patterns—unless, that is, you foster healthy coping mechanisms to help you thrive.

When you're dealing with a trial of some kind—sickness or death of a family member, a difficult job or unemployment, financial problems, depression or anxiety, moving, raising children, chronic disease, upsetting relationships, you name it—you have to learn to accept that many of these concerns are not things you can necessarily "fix" or make go away. What you *can* change is how you respond to and deal with these issues so that you stay on the healthy path you've designed for yourself. Your body will tell you when your emotional health has gone awry, because you may have a change in appetite or weight, GI-related problems (diarrhea, constipation), insomnia, high blood pressure, headaches, racing heart, sexual issues, shortness of breath, or sweating. If you feel persistently lonely or isolated, this can cause poor sleep, severe depression and anxiety, reduced immune and cardiovascular function, and even cognitive decline. For relief, talk about how you feel to a loved one or a professional, focus on the positive, and try to gain perspective. Keep tabs on whether your feelings change for the better, because noticing that the situations that once stressed you out have passed will help your mind let go of the anxiety around them.

Above all, stay aware of your feelings, behaviors, and thought patterns by talking to friends and loved ones. Find techniques that help you be mindful of your stressors and how you deal with them. For example, if you're tempted to reach for alcohol or sugary snacks when you're stressed, find a more positive response, like playing music, drinking herbal tea, or watching a funny TV show. Look for supporters to play on your team, so to speak. Your inner circle should include those who make you a better person (and for whom you do the same). Join social groups to get your mind off your own thoughts, and try to enjoy the people you're around without judging them. Focusing less on yourself and more on others is one of the best ways to find happiness and let go of stress.

Being open to changing your habits and maintaining a positive self-view is important to healthy aging. We all have aspects of our lives that are stressful or that we'd like to improve upon. The best way to handle them is not to dwell upon the negative forces that we cannot control, but instead to focus on positive changes that we can make so that we can live the life we want.

LET'S GET COOKING!

The rest of this book is devoted to delicious recipes that support the mind-healthy guidelines discussed in part I. Because we want you to create a brain-enhancing lifestyle that's easy to maintain, the recipes that follow are simple to prepare and use ingredients widely available at your local grocery store. You don't have to be a bona fide chef to pull them off. It may take some practice, but if you have patience and aren't afraid to make mistakes, you'll be a whiz in no time.

Know, too, that some of these recipes are more time-consuming than others, so be sure to plan ahead using the prep and cook times we've provided. Above all, have fun. Feel free to make these recipes your own. As long as you stay true to the meal's essence and keep the good nutrients in — and unhealthy ingredients as far away from your fork as possible — you'll benefit from every last bite.

Bon appétit to you *and* your mind!

CHAPTER 8

Breakfast

Get into the habit of starting every day with a brain boost. Breakfast is said to be your most important meal, and for good reason. It sets the tone for how you will eat the rest of the day and is the "on switch" for your metabolism. Breakfast is also the easiest meal to plan as a routine, because we typically wake up at the same time every day, and it is usually simple and fast to make. It's important to eat a combination of healthy carbohydrates and protein at breakfast, and it's also a great opportunity to get in a serving of vegetables or leafy greens.

Almond Waffles with Strawberries

Prep time: 10 minutes, plus 30 minutes to chill
Cook time: 15 minutes
Serves 6

These waffles are made with almond flour, which is made by blanching whole almonds, removing the skins, and then finely grinding them. (You can do this yourself in a food processor or look for packaged almond flour in the gluten-free baking section in most supermarkets. Don't confuse almond flour with almond meal, which typically still has the skins and is much coarser.) The result is a slightly nutty, fluffy, nutrient-dense flour. As with many types of batters, the longer this one sits, the better the flours absorb the liquids — and this leads to better taste and texture. I recommend whipping up this recipe the night before both to save time in the morning and to enhance the flavor. Topped with chopped strawberries and pure maple syrup, these waffles are a delicious, brain-healthy treat.

2 cups almond flour

¾ cup spelt flour or whole-wheat flour

2 tablespoons unrefined sugar

1 teaspoon baking soda

¼ teaspoon sea salt

2 cups low-fat milk, plain unsweetened almond milk, or water

¼ cup honey

2 large eggs, lightly beaten

1 teaspoon almond extract or vanilla extract

4 cups chopped strawberries, for serving

¾ cup pure maple syrup, for serving

In a large bowl, combine the almond flour, spelt flour, sugar, baking soda, and salt. Add the milk, honey, eggs, and almond extract and gently mix until everything is fully incorporated. Cover the bowl and refrigerate for at least 30 minutes or up to overnight.

Heat a waffle iron on high. Pour the batter into the waffle iron, making sure not to overfill it. Close the iron and cook for 2 to 4 minutes, or until the waffles are a deep golden brown. Repeat to cook all the waffles. Top the waffles with strawberries and maple syrup.

Chilled Oatmeal and Strawberry-Rhubarb Compote

Prep time: 10 minutes, plus overnight to chill
Cook time: 10 minutes
Serves 4

Chilled oatmeal is a delicious and easy-to-make breakfast that can be prepared at the beginning of the week and refrigerated for when you need to grab and go. The oats take on a nutty, chewy texture. And the berry compote? Divine. Store and serve in mason jars for a pretty presentation.

    3 cups halved strawberries

    2 rhubarb stalks, trimmed and cut into ½-inch pieces, *or* 1 large apple, peeled, cored, and sliced

    3 tablespoons pure maple syrup

    ½ teaspoon ground cinnamon

    2 cups steel-cut oats or quick oats

    2 cups vanilla low-fat Greek yogurt

    4 tablespoons chopped raw walnuts or other nuts, for serving

In a medium saucepan, combine the strawberries, rhubarb, maple syrup, and cinnamon. Bring to a simmer over medium-high heat and cook for 7 to 10 minutes, or until the fruit has become soft and mushy. Remove the compote from the heat and let it cool.

Set out four 1-cup mason jars or small containers with lids. In each, layer one-quarter of the fruit compote, ½ cup of the dry oats, and ½ cup of the yogurt. Cover the jars and refrigerate overnight. Top each serving with 1 tablespoon of chopped walnuts before eating.

Banana Oat Muffins

Prep time: 15 minutes
Cook time: 20 minutes
Serves 12

When you buy muffins from a store or bakery, they are often loaded with sugar—sometimes even more than cupcakes! These muffins have a fraction of the sugar and use whole-grain flours to boost the nutrient level. They are delicious on their own or with a spoonful of creamy natural peanut butter for added protein and healthy fats.

3 ripe bananas, mashed

⅓ cup extra-virgin olive oil

½ cup plain low-fat yogurt

1 large egg, beaten

1 teaspoon pure vanilla extract

¼ cup unrefined sugar

1½ cups spelt flour or whole-wheat flour (or a mix of the two)

1 cup oat bran or oat flour (quick oats ground in a blender or food processor)

1 teaspoon baking soda

1 teaspoon baking powder

1 teaspoon ground cinnamon

½ teaspoon ground cloves

¼ teaspoon ground nutmeg

¼ cup semisweet chocolate chips (optional)

Preheat the oven to 350°F. Lightly grease or spray a muffin tin with olive oil.

In a large bowl, combine the bananas, oil, yogurt, egg, vanilla, and sugar. Gently mix in the flour, oat bran, baking soda, baking powder, cinnamon, cloves, and nutmeg. Stir in the chocolate chips, if desired. Using a ¼-cup measure, scoop the batter into the muffin tin.

Bake the muffins for 18 to 20 minutes, or until an inserted toothpick comes out clean.

Blueberry-Apple Pancakes

Prep time: 10 minutes
Cook time: 10 minutes
Serves 4

Most pancakes are made from white flour. Delicious? Yes. Nutritious? No way. These pancakes are packed with grated apples and oats for a heartier, healthier breakfast. Topped with hot blueberries and a touch of pure maple syrup, they will fill you up with lasting energy.

1½ cups spelt flour or whole-wheat flour

¾ cup quick oats

1 teaspoon baking powder

¼ teaspoon sea salt

1 apple (unpeeled), cored and grated

1 large egg, lightly beaten

2 cups low-fat milk, plain unsweetened almond milk, or water

2 tablespoons sunflower oil

1 tablespoon honey

4 tablespoons soft vegetable-based margarine

Topping

>2 cups blueberries
>
>¼ cup pure maple syrup
>
>2 tablespoons water
>
>1 tablespoon cornstarch

In a large bowl, combine the flour, oats, baking powder, salt, apple, egg, milk, oil, and honey. Stir well to incorporate all the ingredients.

Heat a griddle or large skillet over high heat. Put a tablespoon of margarine in the pan and let it melt. Using a ¼-cup measure, pour the batter onto the griddle, making sure not to crowd the pan. Let the pancakes cook until the bottoms are lightly browned and little bubbles form around then edges, then flip them. Cook until they are lightly browned on the other side, adding more margarine as needed to obtain a golden crust on the pancakes. Repeat until the batter is gone.

While the pancakes are cooking, in a medium saucepan, combine all the topping ingredients. Bring to a simmer over medium heat and cook for 3 to 5 minutes, or until thickened. Pour over the pancakes.

Broccoli and Tomato Frittata

Prep time: 10 minutes
Cook time: 25 minutes
Serves 6

Frittatas make for an easy last-minute dish because you can put just about anything in them. It's a perfect go-to meal when you're strapped for time or low on groceries. This frittata is not only great for breakfast; it makes a delicious dinner served alongside a simple salad or crusty whole-grain bread. The broccoli can be replaced with any leafy green on hand.

2 tablespoons extra-virgin olive oil

1 small yellow onion, diced

1 garlic clove, minced

1 tablespoon minced rosemary

2 cups roughly chopped broccoli florets

½ teaspoon sea salt

½ cup water

3 small Roma tomatoes, diced

8 large eggs

1 cup low-fat milk

¼ cup grated Parmesan cheese

⅛ teaspoon ground black pepper

Preheat the oven to 375°F.

Heat the oil in a large oven-safe skillet over medium heat. Add the onion, garlic, and rosemary and sauté for a minute. Add the broccoli florets and salt and sauté for 2 minutes. Add the water, cover, and cook for 2 minutes, or until slightly tender. Stir in the tomatoes.

In a medium bowl, whisk together the eggs and milk. Add the eggs to the skillet and stir continuously until the eggs start to scramble, about 4 minutes. Top with the Parmesan cheese and pepper. Transfer the skillet to the oven and bake for 15 minutes, or until an inserted knife comes out clean.

Blueberry Smoothie

Prep time: 2 minutes
Serves 1

A berry smoothie is a quick, tasty, nutritious way to start your day. It's great for the mind, the body, and a busy schedule. Add a handful of raw spinach to satisfy your daily greens.

  1 cup fresh or frozen blueberries (frozen is better for texture)

  1 tablespoon natural almond or peanut butter

  2 tablespoons vanilla protein powder

  1 tablespoon ground flaxseed or chia seeds

  1 cup low-fat milk or plain unsweetened almond milk

  Combine all the ingredients in a blender and blend until smooth and creamy.

Spinach Migas

Prep time: 10 minutes
Cook time: 10 minutes
Serves 4

Migas is a popular breakfast throughout Mexico, Spain, and Portugal. This recipe kicks up the nutrient levels with bright green spinach. Feel free to add any other favorite veggie you have on hand.

  ¼ cup extra-virgin olive oil

  1 large whole-grain flour tortilla or 3 small corn tortillas, cut into 3-by-½-inch strips

4 cups roughly chopped spinach

5 large eggs, beaten

½ teaspoon ground cumin

¼ teaspoon sea salt

¼ teaspoon ground black pepper

½ cup favorite salsa

Heat the oil in a large sauté pan over high heat until it is hot but not simmering. Place one tortilla strip in the pan. If it doesn't sizzle immediately, the oil is not hot enough. Once the oil is heated, add the remaining tortilla strips in a single layer and cook for a minute, or until light brown. Flip them over and cook the other side. Transfer to a paper towel–lined plate.

Lower the heat to medium. Add the spinach to the pan, a little at a time until it wilts, and sauté for 2 minutes. Add the eggs, cumin, salt, and pepper. Scramble the eggs for a minute or so. Add the fried tortilla strips and continue scrambling until the eggs are cooked to your desired texture. The tortilla strips should break apart during the scramble. Remove from the heat and stir in the salsa.

Quinoa Breakfast Muffin Cakes

Prep time: 15 minutes
Cook time: 20 minutes
Serves 12

These muffin cakes are denser and moister than your average muffin. Kids love these little treats for breakfast or as a mid-morning or afternoon snack.

1 cup spelt flour or whole-wheat flour

¼ cup oat bran or oat flour (quick oats ground in a blender or food processor)

¼ cup uncooked quinoa, toasted

¼ cup unrefined sugar

1 teaspoon baking powder

1 teaspoon baking soda

1 tablespoon ground cinnamon

¼ teaspoon sea salt

2 carrots, peeled and grated

1 large egg, lightly beaten

¼ cup sunflower oil

1 teaspoon pure vanilla extract

½ cup dried cranberries

¼ cup raw pecans, roughly chopped

Preheat the oven to 350°F. Lightly grease or spray a muffin tin with olive oil.

In a large bowl, combine the flour, oat bran, quinoa, sugar, baking powder, baking soda, cinnamon, and salt. Gently fold in the carrots, egg, oil, vanilla, cranberries, and pecans; be careful not to overmix. Using a ¼-cup measure, scoop the batter into the muffin tin.

Bake the muffins for 18 to 20 minutes, or until an inserted knife comes out clean.

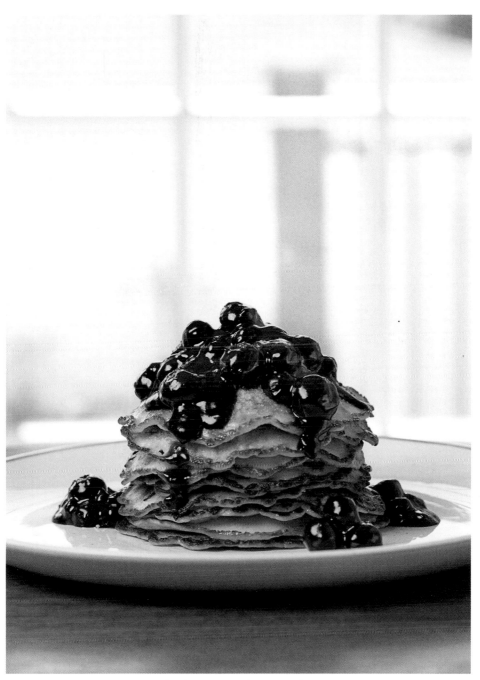

Blueberry-Apple Pancakes

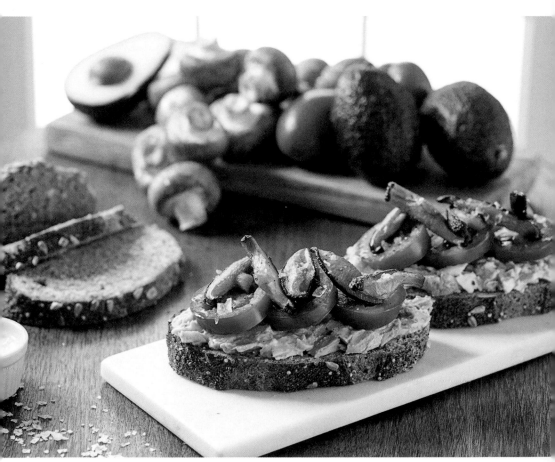

Avocado Toast with Mushrooms and Tomatoes

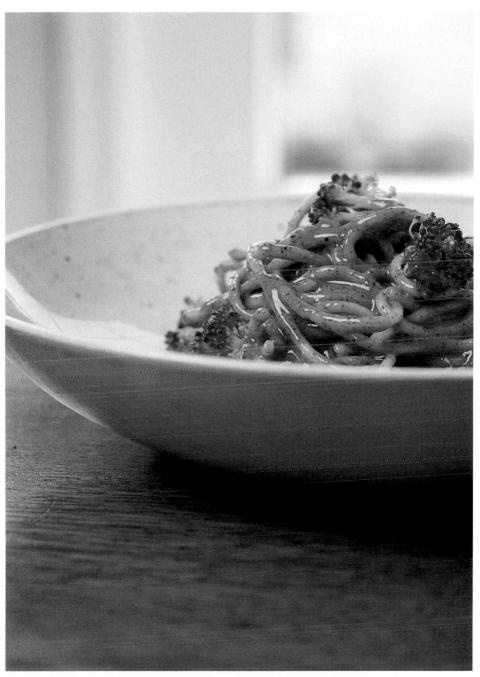

Brown-Rice Spaghetti with Broccoli and Almond Butter Sauce

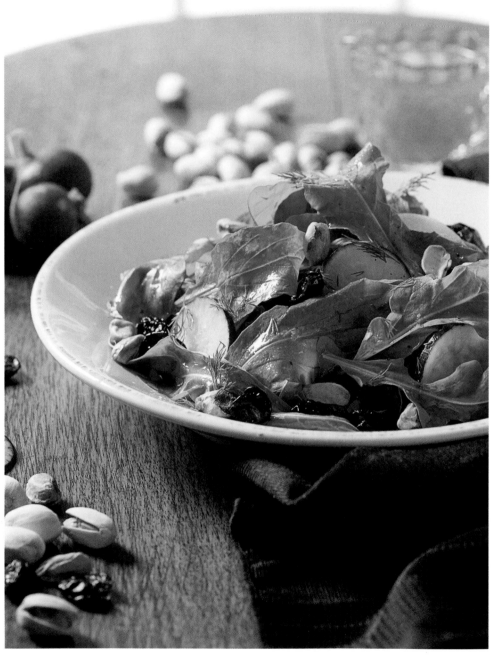

Arugula Salad with Pistachios

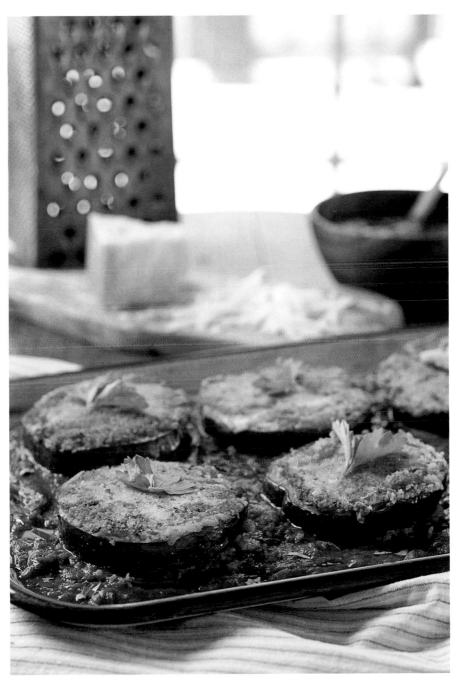

Curried Eggplant Parmesan

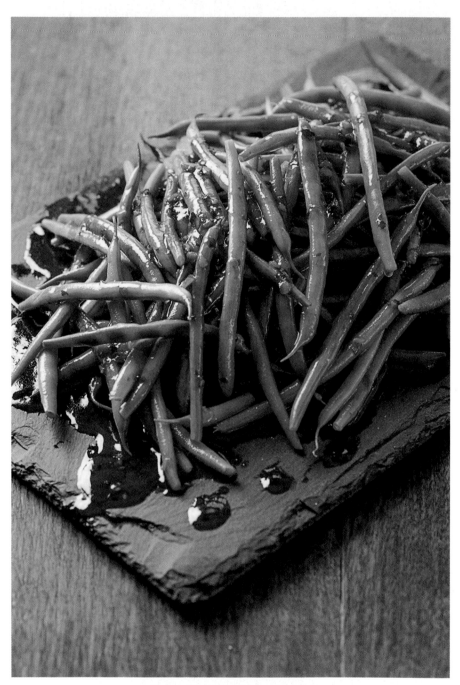

Spicy Honey Green Beans

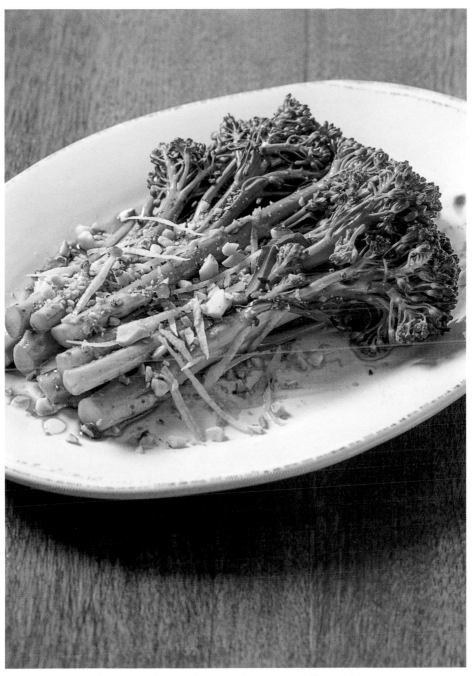

Sautéed Broccolini with Lemony Brazil Nuts

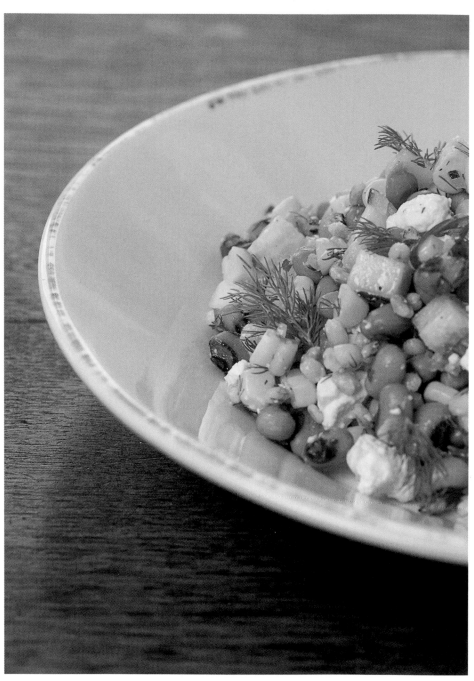

Black-Eyed Pea Summer Salad

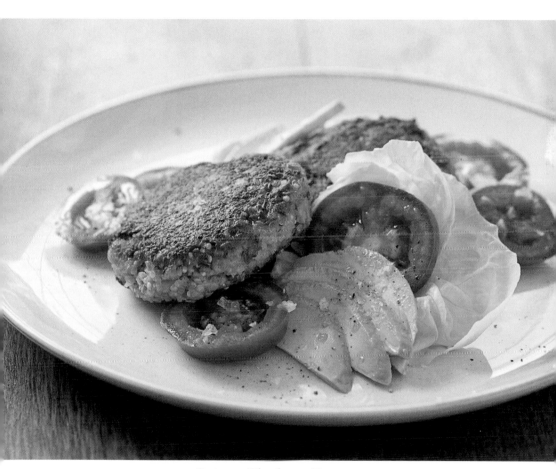

Quinoa-Chickpea Patties

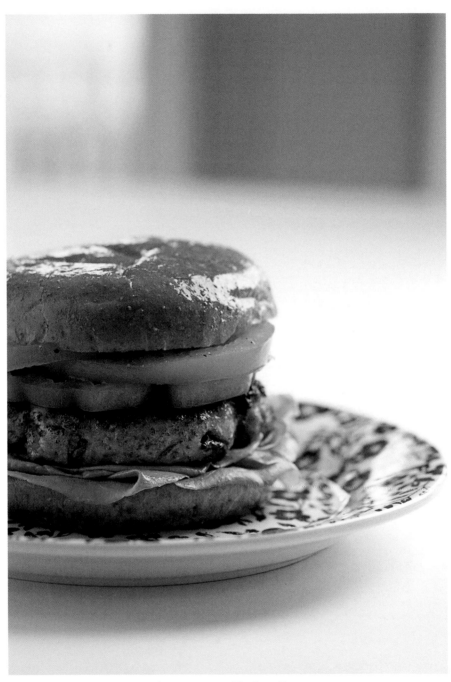

Mediterranean Turkey Burgers

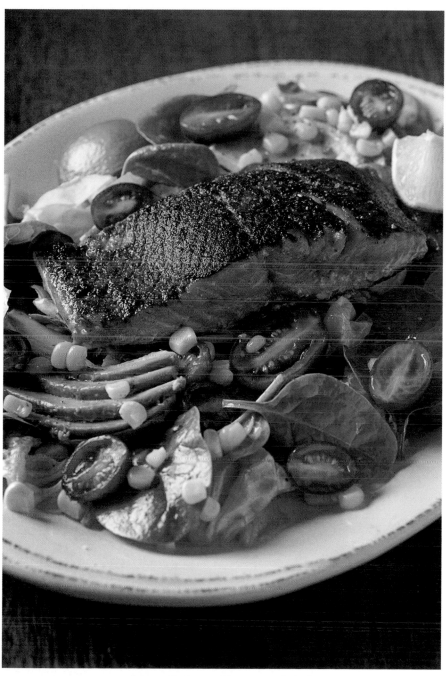

Spicy Salmon Summer Salad

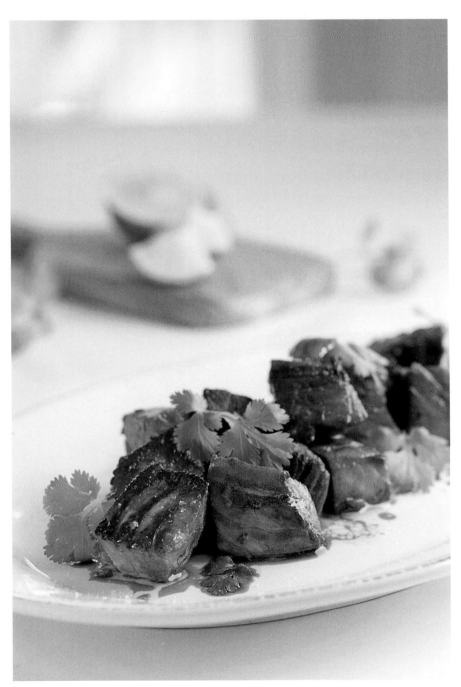

Ahi Tuna Medallions

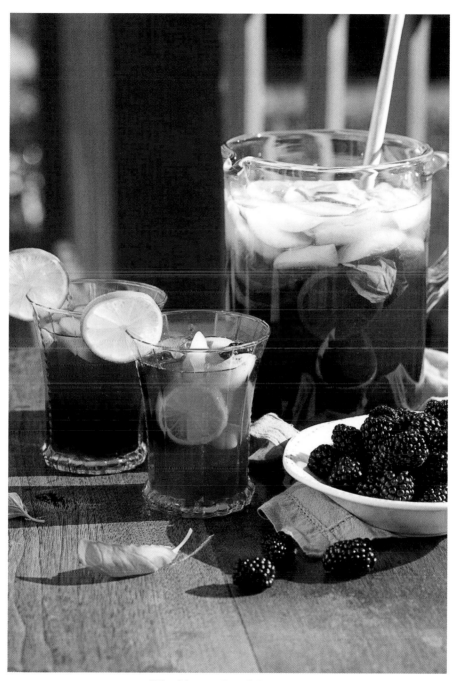

Blackberry-Basil Sangria

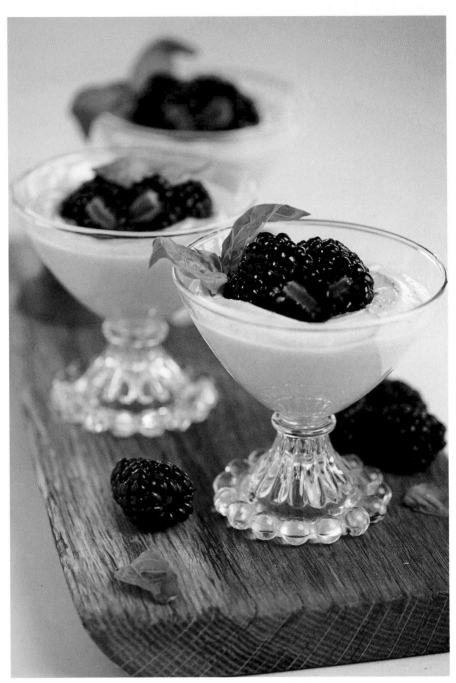

Gingerbread Mousse with Blackberries

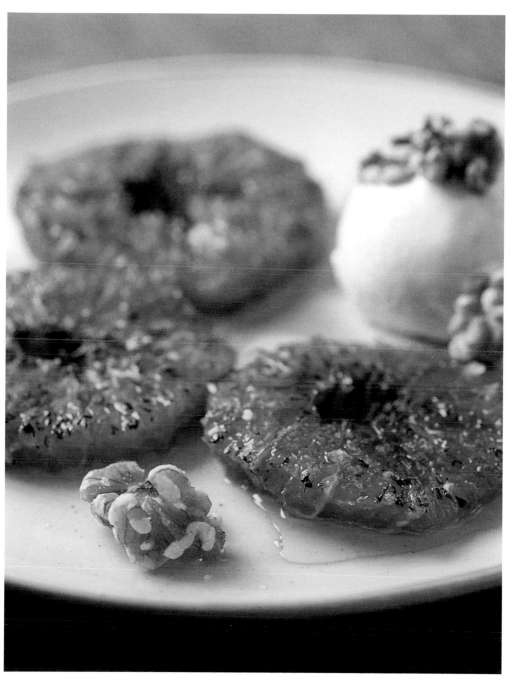

Grilled Pink Grapefruit with Walnuts

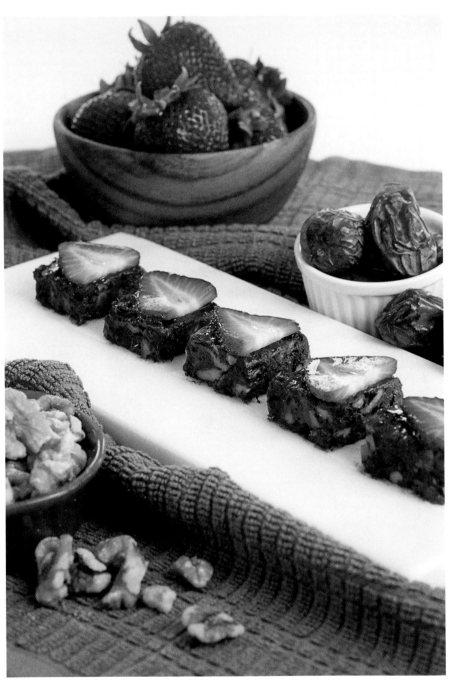

Decadent Brownie Bites

Avocado Toast with Mushrooms and Tomatoes

Prep time: 10 minutes
Cook time: 3 minutes
Serves 2

Avocado toast is packed with flavor and nutrients. I suggest using a crusty artisanal bread from your local baker or farmers' market. For a higher-protein breakfast, add a fried egg on top.

1 teaspoon extra-virgin olive oil

3 ounces shiitake mushrooms, stemmed and sliced

2 slices whole-wheat bread

1 avocado, halved and pitted

2 Roma tomatoes, sliced

¼ teaspoon sea salt

Heat the oil in a medium sauté pan over medium heat. Add the mushrooms and sauté for 2 to 3 minutes, or until golden brown.

While the mushrooms are cooking, toast the bread. Mash and spread half of the avocado onto each slice of toast. Top each slice with tomatoes and mushrooms, then sprinkle with salt.

Spinach and Eggs

Prep time: 7 minutes
Cook time: 7 minutes
Serves 2

This is a favorite go-to breakfast in our home, especially since it gives you your leafy greens first thing in the morning. Feel free to substitute kale for spinach; sautéed mushrooms and tomatoes are a nice addition, too.

- 1 teaspoon extra-virgin olive oil
- 3 cups roughly chopped spinach
- 2 large eggs
- 2 slices whole-wheat bread
- 1 tablespoon goat cheese
- ¼ teaspoon ground black pepper

Heat the oil in a medium sauté pan over medium heat. Add the spinach and sauté for a minute or so, until it's slightly wilted. Transfer the spinach to a plate or push to the side of the pan. Using the same pan, fry the eggs over easy or until your preferred doneness, 2 to 3 minutes.

While the eggs are cooking, toast the bread. Spread each slice with half of the goat cheese, top with spinach and a fried egg, and sprinkle with pepper.

CHAPTER 9

Whole Grains

A diet rich in whole grains has been shown to reduce the risk of type 2 diabetes, heart disease, and obesity, conditions that contribute to impaired brain function. Whole grains are packed with protein, slow-releasing carbohydrates, B vitamins, antioxidants, and trace minerals.

A whole grain contains all parts of the edible grain, including the bran, germ, and endosperm. The whole grain may be used intact, as with barley, or recombined, as with whole-wheat flour, as long as all three parts — the brain, germ, and endosperm — are present in their original proportions. Even if the grain is cracked, crushed, rolled, or extruded, it is still considered a whole grain. Some of the more common whole grains are whole-grain corn, whole oats or oatmeal, brown rice, whole rye, whole-grain barley, millet, wild rice, buckwheat, bulgur, quinoa, whole-wheat flour, spelt flour, and farro.

Intact whole grains such as quinoa and brown rice can be stored in an airtight container in a cool pantry for up to six months. Most whole-grain flours and meals will keep for up to three months in an airtight container in a cool pantry.

Whole grains can be cooked in different ways. They can be

boiled like pasta, steamed like rice, or cooked in liquid over low heat like risotto. Depending on the type of grain, some methods are better than others for optimum taste and texture.

We recommend about three servings of whole grains every day. One serving of whole grains is roughly ½ cup of cooked whole grains or oatmeal, 1 slice of whole-grain bread, ½ cup of cooked whole-grain pasta, or 1 cup of whole-grain ready-to-eat cereal. This is important to remember for portion control. If you eat a sandwich with two slices of bread, you have already eaten two of your three servings for the day. Try to get your servings from different sources of whole grain, not just wheat. If you're new to whole grains and iffy about trying whole-grain pasta, for instance, combine the dish with a medley of other flavors and textures. Eventually your tastes will adapt to the chewier texture—and your body will love the health benefits.

Whole-Wheat Summer Lasagna

Prep time: 20 minutes
Cook time: 1 hour 15 minutes
Serves 6

Lasagna is a comforting, hearty dish. This lasagna uses summer garden vegetables and is lighter in cheese and fat than the traditional version. We also use whole-wheat lasagna noodles to increase the nutrient content. Although this dish is lighter, it is still a more indulgent meal, so should be eaten as such.

> 2 tablespoons extra-virgin olive oil
>
> 1 yellow onion, diced
>
> 1 large zucchini, diced

1 small eggplant, diced

1 large orange bell pepper, seeded and chopped

½ teaspoon sea salt

½ teaspoon ground black pepper

2 (20-ounce) jars tomato sauce

1 (15-ounce) container low-fat ricotta cheese

2 cups shredded low-fat mozzarella cheese

1 large egg, lightly beaten

¼ cup plus 2 tablespoons chopped parsley

12 uncooked whole-wheat lasagna noodles

1 cup grated Parmesan cheese

Preheat the oven to 375°F.

Heat the oil in a large saucepan over medium-high heat. Add the onion and sauté for 1 minute. Add the zucchini, eggplant, bell pepper, ¼ teaspoon of the salt, and ¼ teaspoon of the pepper. Cook for 5 to 7 minutes, or until the vegetables are slightly translucent. Add the tomato sauce, reduce the heat to low, and simmer for 5 minutes.

In a large bowl, combine the ricotta cheese, 1 cup of the mozzarella cheese, the egg, ¼ cup of the parsley, and the remaining ¼ teaspoon salt and ¼ teaspoon pepper. Coat the bottom of a 9-by-13-inch baking dish with about one-quarter of the sauce mixture. Place 4 lasagna noodles on top, then add another quarter of the sauce, followed by half of the ricotta mixture. Add 4 more noodles, then cover with another quarter of the sauce and the remaining ricotta. Place the remaining 4 lasagna noodles on top. Pour on the remaining sauce, scatter the remaining 1 cup mozzarella cheese and the Parmesan cheese over it, and top with the remaining 2 tablespoons of parsley.

Cover the dish with aluminum foil and bake for 40 minutes. Remove the foil and bake for another 15 minutes, or until the pasta is tender and the cheese is bubbly.

Creamy Red Curry Quinoa Risotto

Prep time: 5 minutes
Cook time: 30 minutes
Serves 4

One bite of this creamy, satisfying quinoa risotto, and you'll want to make it every week. You can find red curry paste in the international aisle of most grocery stores. It keeps well in the refrigerator for months after opening, so one jar will last a long time. This dish pairs well with chicken, fish, shrimp, or scallops — or with a heaping serving of your favorite roasted vegetables for a delicious vegetarian meal.

- 1 tablespoon extra-virgin olive oil
- 1 small yellow onion, diced
- 2 tablespoons red curry paste
- 1 cup quinoa, rinsed
- 1¾ cups water or vegetable broth
- ½ cup canned light coconut milk
- ¼ teaspoon sea salt

Heat the oil in a large sauté pan over medium-high heat. Add the onion and sauté for 2 minutes, or until translucent. Add the curry paste and sauté for 1 minute. Add the quinoa and sauté for 1½ minutes, stirring it into the curry paste. Add the water and raise the heat to high to bring to a boil. Reduce the heat to low and cook, stirring occasionally, for 12 to 15 minutes, or until mostly cooked through and slightly chewy. Stir in the coconut milk and salt and cook for another 5 to 7 minutes, or until loose and creamy.

Quinoa, Cherry Tomato, and Feta Salad

Prep time: 10 minutes
Cook time: 20 minutes
Serves 4

Quinoa is packed with protein, fiber, and minerals, and this dish is super easy to make. It's also versatile — you can use any vegetables you have on hand, and it stays fresh for days. Add grilled chicken or steamed salmon for extra protein, and a handful of kale if you'd like.

  1 cup quinoa, rinsed

  2 cups water

  1½ cups cooked chickpeas *or* 1 (15-ounce) can chickpeas, rinsed and drained

  2 cups halved cherry tomatoes

  2 celery stalks, thinly sliced

  ½ cup crumbled low-fat feta cheese

  ¼ cup pumpkin seeds or pine nuts, toasted

  3 scallions, chopped

Dressing

  ⅓ cup extra-virgin olive oil

  3 tablespoons red wine vinegar

  1 tablespoon honey

  ¼ teaspoon sea salt

  ¼ teaspoon ground black pepper

In a medium saucepan, combine the quinoa and water and bring to a boil over high heat. Reduce the heat to low, cover, and cook for 15 to 20 minutes, or until light and fluffy.

While the quinoa is cooking, in a large bowl, combine the chickpeas, tomatoes, celery, feta, pumpkin seeds, and scallions. Add the quinoa once fully cooked.

In a small bowl, whisk together all the dressing ingredients. Pour the dressing over the salad and toss to combine.

Farro and Cremini Mushroom Risotto

Prep time: 15 minutes
Cook time: 45 minutes
Serves 4

Farro is an increasingly popular grain in the wheat family. It is slightly nutty and chewy, which makes for a heartier risotto than traditional Arborio rice. You can use any mushroom you like in this dish, and you can substitute kale for spinach if you prefer.

3 tablespoons extra-virgin olive oil

3 cups thinly sliced cremini mushrooms

½ teaspoon sea salt

¼ teaspoon ground black pepper

6 cups baby spinach leaves

1 shallot, chopped

1 tablespoon chopped fresh rosemary

1½ teaspoons chopped fresh thyme

1 cup farro, rinsed

½ cup dry white wine

6 cups vegetable broth

Heat 2 tablespoons of the oil in a large sauté pan over medium-high heat. Add the mushrooms and sauté for 3 to 5 minutes, or until golden brown. Add the salt and pepper and transfer the mushrooms to a plate.

Reduce the heat to medium, add the spinach, and sauté for 2 to 4 minutes, or until slightly wilted. Transfer the spinach to the plate with the mushrooms.

Add the remaining 1 tablespoon oil. When it is hot, add the shallot, rosemary, and thyme and sauté for 2 minutes. Add the farro and sauté for another 2 minutes. Deglaze with the white wine. Once the liquid has mostly cooked off, about 1½ minutes, add 3 cups of the vegetable broth, reduce the heat to medium-low, and cook, stirring occasionally, for 10 to 15 minutes, or until the liquid has reduced. Add the remaining 3 cups vegetable broth and continue cooking, stirring occasionally, for 15 to 20 minutes, or until the farro is tender. Return the mushrooms and spinach to the pan and stir to combine.

Quinoa and Kale with Toasted Pine Nuts

Prep time: 12 minutes
Cook time: 25 minutes
Serves 4

This dish is pleasingly colorful and equally delicious. It can be made as a side dish but is filling enough to be a light main course. Purple kale, also known as Redbor kale, has a deep magenta color and curly edges. Other varieties of kale can be used for this dish, too.

1 cup red quinoa, rinsed

2 cups water

2 tablespoons extra-virgin olive oil

1 bunch purple kale, stems removed and leaves chopped

2 garlic cloves, minced

¼ teaspoon sea salt

Dressing

2 tablespoons extra-virgin olive oil

2 tablespoons freshly squeezed lemon juice

1 tablespoon honey

¼ teaspoon sea salt

½ cup pine nuts, toasted

In a medium saucepan, combine the quinoa and water and bring to a boil over high heat. Reduce the heat to low, cover, and cook for 15 to 20 minutes, or until light and fluffy.

Heat the oil in a large sauté pan over medium-high heat. Add the kale and cook for 3 to 5 minutes, or until slightly tender. Add the garlic and salt and stir for another 1 to 2 minutes. Remove from the heat and stir in the quinoa.

In a small bowl, whisk together all the dressing ingredients. Pour over the kale and quinoa mixture and stir until it's well incorporated. Transfer to a serving dish. Top with the toasted pine nuts.

Fresh and Light Garlicky Linguine

Prep time: 7 minutes
Cook time: 15 minutes
Serves 4 to 6

Here is a great no-fuss way to prepare whole-grain pasta. It works best with long pastas such as linguine, spaghetti, angel hair, or fettuccine. Pair it with Stuffed Sea Bass (page 218), Baked Shrimp and Scallops (page 212), or any salmon dish.

1 pound whole-wheat linguine

4 tablespoons extra-virgin olive oil

1 shallot, chopped

2 garlic cloves, chopped

⅓ cup dry white wine

Juice of ½ lemon

⅔ cup chopped fresh parsley

¼ teaspoon sea salt

¼ teaspoon ground black pepper

Bring a large pot of water to a boil over high heat. Add the linguine and cook for 8 minutes, or until the pasta is mostly cooked but still has a slight bite (al dente). Before draining, reserve 1 cup of the cooking water.

Heat 1 tablespoon of the oil in a large sauté pan over medium heat. Add the shallot and garlic and sauté for 1 to 1½ minutes. Deglaze with the white wine. Let the liquid reduce by half, about 1 minute.

Reduce the heat to low and add the cooked linguine and the remaining 3 tablespoons oil. Stir to combine. Add ½ to 1 cup of the pasta cooking water as needed to achieve the desired consistency. Add the lemon juice, parsley, salt, and pepper.

Skinny Taco Bowls

Prep time: 15 minutes
Cook time: 20 minutes
Serves 6

Though this meal could easily be categorized under poultry, legumes, or vegetables, we especially love its whole-grain appeal. A great alternative to eating large servings of grains is to add a couple of spoonfuls of your favorite whole grains to salads and soups. You can easily substitute brown rice for quinoa in this recipe, and it will be just as tasty. For extra flavor, cook your whole grains in low-sodium vegetable or chicken broth.

1 cup red quinoa, rinsed

2¼ cups water

2 tablespoons extra-virgin olive oil

1 small yellow onion, diced

1 tablespoon dried minced onion

1 teaspoon garlic salt

1 teaspoon ground cumin

½ teaspoon smoked paprika

1 pound lean ground turkey

1 (15-ounce) can black beans, rinsed and drained

1 cup fresh or thawed frozen corn

1 large orange bell pepper, seeded and chopped

½ cup chopped fresh cilantro

Dressing

¼ cup extra-virgin olive oil

Juice of 1 lime

1 tablespoon honey

1 avocado, peeled, pitted, and sliced

Combine the quinoa and 2 cups of the water in a medium saucepan and bring to a boil over high heat. Reduce the heat to low, cover, and cook for 15 to 20 minutes, or until light and fluffy.

While the quinoa is cooking, heat the oil in another medium saucepan over medium-high heat. Add the diced onion and sauté for 2 minutes. Add the dried minced onion, garlic salt, cumin, and smoked paprika and sauté for 1 minute. Add the ground turkey and brown for 5 minutes, breaking up the meat into small chunks. Add the remaining ¼ cup water, reduce the heat to medium-low, and cook for another 5 to 7 minutes, or until the turkey is fully cooked through. Remove from the heat.

In a large bowl, toss together the quinoa, black beans, corn, bell pepper, and cilantro. Add the turkey mixture. In a small bowl, whisk together all the dressing ingredients. Pour over the salad and toss to combine. Top with the avocado slices.

Brown-Rice Spaghetti with Broccoli and Almond Butter Sauce

Prep time: 10 minutes
Cook time: 20 minutes
Serves 5

Alternatives for wheat pasta have become increasingly popular due to gluten and wheat sensitivities. Brown-rice spaghetti provides the health benefits of whole grains and still delivers the flavor and texture you expect from traditional white rice noodles, which contain fewer nutrients. This dish tastes delicious served cold the next day.

1 pound brown-rice spaghetti

Almond Butter Sauce

¾ cup almond butter

⅔ cup low-sodium soy sauce or tamari

Juice of 2 limes

2 tablespoons grated fresh ginger

2 tablespoons sunflower oil

4 cups small broccoli florets

1 cup water

Bring a large pot of water to a boil over high heat. Add the spaghetti and cook for 6 to 8 minutes, or until the pasta is mostly cooked but still has a slight bite (al dente). Immediately drain and rinse under very cold water for 2 minutes to stop the cooking process and to prevent the noodles from sticking together.

In a medium bowl, whisk together all the sauce ingredients.

Heat the oil in a wok or large sauté pan over medium-high heat. Add the broccoli florets and sauté for 5 minutes. Add the water, reduce the heat to medium, and cover. Steam the broccoli until it is bright green and has a slight bite, about 6 minutes. Add the noodles and sauce to the wok and stir to combine. Cook for 2 minutes to heat through.

Sweet Corn Tacos

Prep time: 20 minutes
Cook time: 20 minutes
Serves 4 to 6

Compared to flour tortillas, corn tortillas are higher in fiber and magnesium and lower in sugar and sodium. They are also smaller, so they come with built-in portion control, and are gluten-free. These tacos combine a rainbow of flavors, and the leftovers taste even better.

12 corn tortillas

2 ears corn

2 avocados, peeled, pitted, and cut into cubes

1 jalapeño, seeded if desired and minced

½ cup finely chopped pitted dates

¼ cup chopped fresh cilantro

2 tablespoons chopped fresh basil

½ cup crumbled low-fat feta cheese

Juice of 2 limes

¼ teaspoon ground black pepper

1 tablespoon extra-virgin olive oil

½ small white onion, diced

1 (15-ounce) can black beans, rinsed and drained

¼ cup water

1 teaspoon ground cumin

½ teaspoon garlic powder

On a microwave-safe plate, microwave the corn tortillas in batches on high for 2 to 4 minutes, or until soft.

Remove any dry outer husks or silks poking out of the tops of the ears of corn, but don't husk them. Microwave the ears of corn, one at a time, for 4 minutes on high. Once they're cool enough to handle, remove the husk and silks. Hold each ear of corn vertically on a cutting board and cut off the kernels. Transfer the kernels to a medium bowl. Add the avocados, jalapeño, dates, cilantro, basil, feta cheese, lime juice, and black pepper. Gently stir together.

Heat the oil in a medium sauté pan over medium heat. Add the onion and sauté for 2 to 4 minutes, or until slightly translucent. Add the black beans, water, cumin, and garlic powder and cook for another 4 minutes.

To assemble, place 2 or 3 corn tortillas on each plate. Scoop a heaping spoonful of the black bean mixture in the center of each tortilla. Top with a heaping spoonful of the corn mixture. Fold in half to eat.

Wild Rice with Fire-Roasted Tomatoes

Prep time: 5 minutes
Cook time: 1 hour
Serves 4

Wild rice can improve heart health and stimulate repair throughout the body. It is loaded with essential minerals and nutrients that are great for the brain. It's both nutty and sweet, and can be found in various wild rice blends or mixed wild rice. This dish is a great way to start incorporating the earthier flavor of wild rice into your repertoire. It takes a while to cook, but you don't need to fuss over it. This recipe brings heat and heartiness to a meal and can stand alone as a vegetarian dish. Want to add a little pizzazz? Roast up halved acorn squash to use as bowls for your wild rice.

2 tablespoons extra-virgin olive oil

1 cup mixed wild rice

1 teaspoon garlic powder

½ teaspoon chili powder

3 cups vegetable broth

1 (15-ounce) can fire-roasted tomatoes

1 (15-ounce) can black beans, rinsed and drained

½ cup chopped fresh cilantro

Heat the oil in a large saucepan over medium-high heat. Add the wild rice and sauté for 3 minutes. Stir in the garlic powder and chili powder and sauté for 1½ minutes. Add the broth, raise the heat to high, and bring to a boil. Reduce the heat to medium-low and stir in the fire-roasted tomatoes with their juice. Cover and simmer for 45 minutes. Add the beans, cover, and cook for another 15 minutes, or until the rice is tender. Top with the cilantro.

CHAPTER 10

Leafy Greens

Leafy green vegetables are nutritional powerhouses filled with vitamins, minerals, and phytonutrients. This abundant group of vegetables is inexpensive and can be found year-round in grocery stores. Common leafy green vegetables include romaine lettuce, green leaf lettuce, butterhead lettuce (the most familiar varieties are Boston and Bibb), arugula, kale, mustard greens, collard greens, Swiss chard, and spinach.

When picking out leafy greens, look for a bright green color and no wilted leaves. Leafy greens retain their crispness for up to a week when properly stored in the refrigerator.

Leafy greens can be prepared in many different ways. They can be eaten raw, sautéed, baked, braised, blanched, or roasted. Be careful when cooking them, as some varieties can easily become wilted and drab when overcooked. The best way to maintain the bright color of green vegetables (not just leafy greens) is to avoid prolonged heat and acid. So if you are cooking them to be served at a later time, remove them from the heat while still bright and submerge them in an ice bath to cool immediately; otherwise serve them hot immediately after cooking. When adding a salad dressing with an acid like vinegar, do so just before serving so as to not wilt the greens.

Spinach Salad with Peanut Dressing

Prep time: 15 minutes
Cook time: 20 minutes
Serves 4

With its variety of textures, this tasty, hearty spinach salad is a real crowd pleaser. It's great on its own or pairs well with Ahi Tuna Medallions (page 223).

½ cup quinoa, rinsed

1 cup water

4 ounces whole-wheat spaghetti

6 cups baby spinach

1 cucumber, diced

1 orange bell pepper, seeded and chopped

Dressing

1½ tablespoons honey

1 tablespoon white wine vinegar

1 tablespoon low-sodium soy sauce or tamari

1 tablespoon peanut butter

⅓ cup extra-virgin olive oil

In a small saucepan, combine the quinoa and water and bring to a boil over high heat. Reduce the heat to low, cover, and cook for 15 to 20 minutes, or until light and fluffy.

While the quinoa is cooking, bring a medium pot of water to a boil over high heat. Add the spaghetti and cook for 8 minutes, or until the pasta is mostly cooked but still has a slight bite (al dente). Drain and rinse under cold water.

In a large bowl, combine the quinoa, spaghetti, spinach, cucumber, and bell pepper.

In a small bowl, whisk together the honey, vinegar, soy sauce, and peanut butter. Slowly whisk in the oil. Pour over the salad and lightly toss.

Swiss Chard and Sun-Dried Tomato Lasagna

Prep time: 15 minutes
Cook time: 1 hour
Serves 8

This lasagna includes the perfect balance of sweet sun-dried tomatoes and hearty Swiss chard. Add portobello mushrooms or natural turkey sausage for a meatier dish that is packed with flavor.

2 tablespoons extra-virgin olive oil

1 bunch Swiss chard, finely chopped (stems included)

1 garlic clove, chopped

1 cup oil-packed sun-dried tomatoes, roughly chopped

1 (20-ounce) jar tomato sauce

½ cup water

1 (15-ounce) container low-fat ricotta cheese

1 large egg, lightly beaten

1 cup grated Parmesan cheese

¾ cup chopped fresh parsley

¼ teaspoon sea salt

¼ teaspoon ground black pepper

8 uncooked whole-wheat lasagna noodles

Preheat the oven to 375°F.

Heat the oil in a large sauté pan over medium-high heat. Add the Swiss chard and sauté for 3 minutes. Add the garlic and sauté for another 30 seconds. Add the sun-dried tomatoes, tomato sauce, and water and stir to combine. Simmer for 6 minutes. Remove from the heat.

In a large bowl, combine the ricotta cheese, egg, ½ cup of the Parmesan cheese, ½ cup of the parsley, and the salt and pepper. Coat the bottom of a 9-by-11-inch baking dish with about one-third of the sauce. Place 4 lasagna noodles on top, then add another third of the sauce, followed by the ricotta mixture. Add 4 more noodles and cover with the remaining sauce. Top with the remaining ½ cup Parmesan cheese and ¼ cup parsley.

Cover the dish with aluminum foil and bake for 30 minutes. Remove the foil and bake for another 15 to 20 minutes, or until the pasta is tender and the cheese is melted and slightly golden. Cool for 5 to 10 minutes before serving.

Butternut Squash and Kale Gratin

Prep time: 20 minutes
Cook time: 50 minutes
Serves 6

Smooth and sweet butternut squash, slightly bitter sautéed kale, and fluffy ricotta make for a highly textured dish that speaks to all your cravings.

1 large butternut squash

3 tablespoons extra-virgin olive oil

1 bunch kale, stems removed and leaves chopped

¼ teaspoon sea salt

¼ teaspoon chili powder

⅛ teaspoon ground nutmeg

1 (15-ounce) container low-fat ricotta cheese

1 large egg, beaten

¼ cup plus 2 tablespoons grated Parmesan cheese

Preheat the oven to 375°F. Lightly grease or spray a 9-by-11-inch baking dish with olive oil.

Peel the butternut squash. Cut the neck into ½-inch-thick slices; reserve the bulb for another use.

Heat 2 tablespoons of the oil in a large sauté pan over medium heat. Add the kale and sauté for 5 minutes. Stir in the salt, chili powder, and nutmeg and sauté for another 2 minutes. Remove from the heat.

In a large bowl, combine the ricotta cheese, egg, and ¼ cup of the Parmesan cheese. Place half of the butternut squash slices in a single layer in the baking dish. Spoon the ricotta mixture over the butternut squash and spread evenly. Layer the kale over the ricotta mixture and spread evenly. Place the remaining butternut squash slices in a single layer on top of the kale. Top with the remaining 2 tablespoons Parmesan cheese and drizzle on the remaining 1 tablespoon olive oil.

Cover the dish with aluminum foil and bake for 30 minutes. Remove the foil and bake for another 10 to 15 minutes. Test for doneness by inserting a knife all the way through the layers. The butternut squash should be tender and the knife should insert easily.

Kale Caesar Salad

Prep time: 10 minutes
Cook time: 3 minutes
Serves 4 to 6

Caesar salad is a favorite go-to in restaurants for its creamy dressing and crunchy leaves. This version adds curly kale for a dark leafy green punch. The Caesar dressing is made with Greek yogurt and, with homemade croutons, the salad hits all the right notes.

> 3 tablespoons extra-virgin olive oil
>
> 2 slices pumpernickel bread, cut into ½-inch cubes
>
> ¼ teaspoon sea salt

Dressing

> ½ cup low-fat plain Greek yogurt
>
> ¼ cup extra-virgin olive oil
>
> 3 tablespoons freshly squeezed lemon juice
>
> 2 teaspoons Dijon mustard
>
> 1 teaspoon Worcestershire sauce
>
> ¼ teaspoon minced garlic
>
> ¼ teaspoon sea salt
>
> ¼ teaspoon ground black pepper

> 1 bunch curly kale, stems removed and leaves shredded
>
> 2 cups chopped romaine lettuce

Heat the oil in a medium sauté pan over medium heat. Add the bread cubes and cook for 1 to 2 minutes. Toss them gently in the pan and cook for another 1 to 2 minutes, or until golden brown. Transfer them to a paper towel–lined plate and sprinkle with the salt.

In a small bowl, whisk together all the dressing ingredients until they're fully incorporated. Combine the kale and romaine in a large salad bowl. Pour the dressing over the greens and toss to combine. Top with the croutons.

Kale and Spinach Spanakopita

Prep time: 25 minutes
Cook time: 25 minutes
Serves 6

Spanakopita is a delicious Greek dish that's typically loaded with butter and fat. This version uses extra-virgin olive oil and a light layer of phyllo dough to keep calories in check but flavor abundant.

- 2 tablespoons extra-virgin olive oil, plus about ¼ cup more for brushing
- 1 bunch kale, stems removed and leaves roughly chopped
- 1 pound spinach, roughly chopped
- 2 tablespoons minced garlic
- ½ teaspoon chili powder
- ¼ teaspoon ground nutmeg
- ¼ teaspoon sea salt
- ¼ teaspoon ground black pepper
- 1 cup crumbled light feta cheese
- ¼ cup plus 2 tablespoons grated Parmesan cheese
- 12 phyllo dough sheets

Preheat the oven to 375°F.

Heat 2 tablespoons of the oil in a large sauté pan over medium-high heat. Add the kale and cook for 5 minutes, stirring frequently. Push the kale to the side of the pan and add the spinach in batches, while it cooks down. Sauté the spinach for 3 minutes, or until it's just wilted. Add the garlic, chili powder, nutmeg, salt, and pepper and stir the greens together. Reduce the heat to low. Add the feta and 2 tablespoons of the Parmesan cheese. Mix for 30 seconds, then turn off the heat.

Place one sheet of phyllo dough in a 9-by-11-inch baking dish. Brush it lightly with olive oil, using either a pastry brush or your fingertips. Add five more sheets of phyllo, brushing each with oil. Spoon the kale and spinach mixture on top of the phyllo, spreading it evenly. Layer on the remaining six sheets of phyllo, brushing each layer with oil, including the top sheet. Top the phyllo with the remaining ¼ cup Parmesan cheese.

Bake for 15 minutes, or until golden brown.

Arugula Salad with Pistachios

Prep time: 10 minutes
Serves 4

This beautiful salad features a delicious medley of flavors. It can accompany just about any protein or veggie burger.

6 cups arugula

4 radishes, thinly sliced

½ cup shelled pistachios

⅓ cup dried cherries or cranberries

¼ cup chopped fresh dill

Dressing

> 2 tablespoons freshly squeezed orange juice
>
> 1 tablespoon red wine vinegar
>
> 1 tablespoon honey
>
> 1 tablespoon grated orange zest
>
> ¼ cup extra-virgin olive oil

In a salad bowl, layer the arugula, radish slices, pistachios, dried cherries, and dill. In a small bowl, whisk together the orange juice, vinegar, honey, and orange zest. Slowly whisk in the oil. Pour the dressing over the salad and lightly toss.

Lemony Spinach Salad

Prep time: 10 minutes
Serves 6

Spinach salads are a convenient, accessible way to get in your daily serving of greens. I love this salad because the thinly sliced spinach leaves make it simple to mix—and eat! It's great on its own or as a base for whatever vegetables you want to throw in. Add chicken, fish, or your favorite grain or legume to make a more filling meal.

> 8 cups spinach chiffonade (thin ribbons)
>
> 1 large orange bell pepper, seeded and thinly sliced
>
> 1 cucumber, diced
>
> ½ cup crumbled light feta cheese

Dressing

2 tablespoons freshly squeezed lemon juice

1 tablespoon honey

1½ teaspoons Dijon mustard

1 teaspoon grated lemon zest

¼ cup extra-virgin olive oil

In a large salad bowl, combine the spinach, pepper, cucumber, and feta cheese. In a small bowl, whisk together the lemon juice, honey, Dijon, and lemon zest. Slowly whisk in the oil until it's well incorporated. Pour over the salad and toss.

Super Green Stir-Fry

Prep time: 10 minutes
Cook time: 10 minutes
Serves 4

When preparing a stir-fry, be sure to chop all your veggies and make your sauce ahead of time so it can all be added to the pan without delay. The idea is to cook the veggies quickly to keep them crisp and bright. This dish is perfect for a light and flavorful midweek dinner. Add chicken or shrimp for protein and serve with your favorite rice or quinoa.

Sauce

⅓ cup chicken broth, vegetable broth, or water

⅓ cup low-sodium soy sauce or tamari

Juice of ½ lime

1 teaspoon oyster sauce

1 teaspoon red chili paste

3 tablespoons grated fresh ginger

1 garlic clove, minced

Stir-Fry

¼ cup sunflower oil

1 small white onion, diced

4 cups small broccoli florets

2 cups chopped bok choy

2 cups snap peas, ends trimmed

In a small bowl, whisk together all the sauce ingredients and set aside.

Heat the oil in a wok or large sauté pan over high heat. Add the onion, broccoli, bok choy, and snap peas. Stirring frequently, cook the vegetables for 4 to 7 minutes, or until they're bright green. Add the sauce and stir. Cover and reduce the heat to medium-low. Cook the vegetables for another 2 to 5 minutes, or until they're cooked through but still slightly crunchy.

Sautéed Spinach

Prep time: 5 minutes
Cook time: 2 to 3 minutes
Serves 2

Use this simple recipe as a starting point for any meal you like. Sautéed spinach is great when it's tossed into a pasta dish, scrambled with an egg, added to a hot sandwich or soup, or folded into a stir-fry.

1 tablespoon extra-virgin olive oil

6 cups chopped spinach

¼ teaspoon sea salt

¼ teaspoon ground black pepper

1 teaspoon freshly squeezed lemon juice

Heat the oil in a medium sauté pan over medium heat. Add the spinach and cook, stirring frequently, for 2 minutes, or until it's slightly wilted and bright green. Remove from the heat. Stir in the salt, pepper, and lemon juice.

Sweet Potato Cakes with Braised Collard Greens

Prep time: 15 minutes, plus 30 minutes to chill
Cook time: 45 minutes
Serves 4

Collards are slightly sweet, tender greens that just happen to be loaded with essential vitamins and minerals. You can find them in the grocery store almost year-round. This recipe is layered with flavors and textures and showcases how easy these versatile greens are to cook.

½ cup quinoa, rinsed

1 cup water

1 large sweet potato

1 large egg, lightly beaten

¼ cup orange juice

¼ cup whole-wheat breadcrumbs

½ teaspoon chili powder

½ teaspoon sea salt

4 to 5 tablespoons extra-virgin olive oil

1 bunch collard greens, stems removed and leaves roughly
   chopped

1 garlic clove, minced

1 (15-ounce) can sliced peaches in juice (not syrup), undrained

In a small saucepan, combine the quinoa and water and bring to
a boil over high heat. Reduce the heat to low, cover, and cook for 15
to 20 minutes, or until light and fluffy. Remove from the heat and set
aside to cool.

While the quinoa is cooling, use a knife to lightly pierce the skin
of the sweet potato about ten times on all sides. Microwave the
sweet potato on high for 3 minutes, rotate in the microwave, and
cook for another 3 minutes, or until the sweet potato is soft when a
knife is inserted. Once it is cool enough to handle, peel off the skin. In
a large bowl, mash the sweet potato with a fork until mostly creamy.
Add the quinoa, egg, orange juice, breadcrumbs, chili powder, and
¼ teaspoon of the salt and mix well. Form the mixture into eight
patties. Place on a plate, cover, and refrigerate for 30 minutes.

Heat 2 tablespoons of the oil in a large sauté pan over medium-
high heat. Add the collard greens and sauté for 5 minutes, stirring
frequently. Add the garlic and sauté for 2 minutes. Add the peaches
with their juice, reduce the heat to medium-low, and cook for 10
minutes. Add the remaining ¼ teaspoon salt and stir. Transfer the
collard greens to a serving dish.

In the same pan, heat another 2 tablespoons oil over medium-
high heat. Add four of the patties, making sure not to crowd the pan.
Cook for 2 to 3 minutes per side, or until a golden crust forms. Place
the cooked patties on top of the collard greens. Repeat with the
remaining four patties, adding the remaining 1 tablespoon oil to the
pan if necessary.

CHAPTER 11

Other Vegetables

To help prevent cognitive decline and dementias like Alzheimer's disease, you'll want to eat at least one serving of vegetables other than leafy greens every day. Choose any vegetable you wish, but as you know, the more variety you eat, the more nutrients you take in. One of the advantages of loading your diet with vegetables is that they're a cost-effective way to add flavor, especially if you eat local produce when it's in season. And if you eat vegetables seasonally, you'll be getting more nutritional benefits as well as more flavor—it's worth the wait!

Cooking vegetables properly might seem tricky, but like anything else, the more you do it, the better you'll be at it. The ideal texture for flavor, nutrient level, and doneness is crisp but tender with a bright, vibrant color. Here are a few tips:

- Try to cut vegetables into uniform shapes to ensure even cooking.

- Whenever possible, cook your vegetables just before serving them to preserve the best flavor and texture. Avoid having to reheat them.

- Green vegetables will wilt with heat and acid. Keep them bright by submerging them in an ice bath immediately after cooking them. And don't add an acid such as vinegar until just before serving.

- When cooking orange, red, purple, and white vegetables — think carrots, sweet potatoes, purple cabbage, beets, and cauliflower — add a squeeze of lemon or a sprinkle of vinegar (or another acid) to keep the colors bright and vibrant.

- Many of the fat-soluble vitamins are found in vegetables, so they are best consumed with a source of fat such as olive oil, vegetable oil, avocados, nuts, or fatty fish for optimal nutrient absorption.

Curried Eggplant Parmesan

Prep time: 15 minutes
Cook time: 30 minutes
Serves 4

This is not your typical eggplant parm. With a fraction of the fat, plus an easy and delicious method for getting the breadcrumbs to stick (hello, hummus!), this delicious meal will become a family favorite. Pair it with Tangy Roasted Cauliflower (page 187) or a light salad for a satisfying dinner.

1 (15-ounce) jar tomato sauce

2 purple eggplants

1½ cups panko breadcrumbs (preferably whole wheat)

2 tablespoons yellow curry powder

¼ teaspoon sea salt

1 cup hummus

½ cup grated Parmesan cheese

4 to 6 tablespoons extra-virgin olive oil

Preheat the oven to 400°F.

Line a 9-by-13-inch baking dish with aluminum foil, and pour in the tomato sauce to coat the entire bottom. Set aside.

Trim the eggplants and cut into ½-inch-thick rounds, aiming to get 4 to 6 slices per eggplant. On a large plate, mix the panko, curry powder, and salt. One at a time, spread a generous layer of hummus on both sides of each eggplant slice. Dredge the slices gently in the breadcrumb mix to make sure that both sides are evenly coated. Sprinkle one side of the eggplant slices with Parmesan cheese and gently press down so the cheese sticks.

Heat 2 to 3 tablespoons of the oil in a large sauté pan over medium-high heat. Add a few eggplant slices, Parmesan-cheese-side down, making sure not to crowd the pan. Cook for 2 to 4 minutes, or until a golden crust forms on the bottom, then flip and cook for another 2 to 4 minutes. Transfer the eggplant slices to the sauce in the baking dish, Parmesan-cheese-side up. Add more oil to the sauté pan as needed and repeat until all the eggplant slices are cooked and transferred to the baking dish.

Bake for 15 to 20 minutes, or until the eggplant is tender.

Spicy Honey Green Beans

Prep time: 5 minutes

Cook time: 10 minutes

Serves 4

Try these crunchy green beans for a slightly sweet, slightly spicy addition to your meals. They take very little time to prepare and cook and are great cold, too. This dish pairs nicely with steamed salmon.

    2 tablespoons toasted sesame oil

    2 pounds French green beans (haricots verts)

    ½ cup water

    2 tablespoons honey

    1 teaspoon red chili paste

Heat the oil in a large sauté pan over medium-high heat. Add the green beans and sauté for 2 to 4 minutes, or until the beans are bright green but still crunchy. Add the water, cover, and steam for 4 to 6 minutes, or until the green beans are still bright green and slightly tender.

In a small bowl, whisk together the honey and red chili paste. Add the mixture to the green beans in the pan and toss gently until all the green beans are coated. Serve immediately.

Roasted Asparagus and Mushrooms with Goat Cheese

Prep time: 10 minutes
Cook time: 15 minutes
Serves 4

Roasted vegetables are one of the simplest and most delicious side dishes. Use your favorite mushrooms—just be sure to cut larger varieties like portobellos into smaller pieces. You can easily buy already-reduced balsamic vinegar in most grocery stores, and it's great to have on hand to add to salads, serve on top of fish and chicken, or drizzle, as in this recipe, over hot roasted vegetables.

1 pound asparagus, trimmed

2 pounds shiitake mushrooms, stems removed

2 tablespoons extra-virgin olive oil

¼ teaspoon sea salt

¼ cup balsamic vinegar

1 teaspoon honey

¼ cup crumbled goat cheese

Preheat the oven to 375°F. Line a large rimmed baking sheet with aluminum foil.

Put the asparagus and mushrooms on the baking sheet. Add the oil and salt and toss gently, then spread out in a single layer. Roast for 15 minutes.

Meanwhile, in a small microwaveable bowl, combine the balsamic vinegar and honey. Microwave in 30-second intervals, stirring in between. Continue for about 3 minutes, or until the vinegar is reduced to a thick, syrupy consistency.

Transfer the roasted vegetables to a serving plate. Using a spoon, drizzle the balsamic reduction over the vegetables in a light, thin layer. Top with the goat cheese and serve hot.

Sweet Potato Rounds with Roasted Kale

Prep time: 10 minutes
Cook time: 20 minutes
Serves 6

Sweet potatoes and kale are a match made in nutritional heaven, but if you don't have kale, these sweet potato rounds are terrific on their own. This dish pairs well with just about any protein, from steamed salmon to Baked Shrimp and Scallops (page 212).

1½ teaspoons ground cumin

1 teaspoon garlic powder

1 teaspoon paprika

½ teaspoon cayenne pepper

½ teaspoon sea salt

2 large sweet potatoes, scrubbed and cut into ½-inch-thick rounds

4 tablespoons extra-virgin olive oil

1 bunch kale, stems removed and leaves roughly torn

Preheat the oven to 400°F. Line two rimmed baking sheets with aluminum foil.

In a small bowl, combine the cumin, garlic powder, paprika, cayenne, and ¼ teaspoon of the salt. In a large bowl, toss the sweet potato slices with 2 tablespoons of the oil. Add the spice mixture to the bowl and mix until all the slices are coated. Place the sweet potato slices on one of the baking sheets in a mostly single layer; it's okay if they're slightly overlapping.

Put the kale on the other baking sheet. Drizzle with the remaining 2 tablespoons oil and ¼ teaspoon salt. Using your hands, toss the kale so the oil is well distributed. Spread the kale evenly on the baking sheet so there is not too much overlap.

Put both baking sheets in the oven. Bake the sweet potatoes for 10 minutes, then flip the slices and bake for another 10 minutes. They should be golden and tender when tested with a knife. Bake the kale for 10 minutes, then gently mix and bake for another 5 minutes, or until just slightly crisp. Transfer the sweet potato rounds to a plate and top with the kale.

Tangy Roasted Cauliflower

Prep time: 15 minutes
Cooke time: 25 minutes
Serves 4

If you know someone who doesn't like cauliflower, this slightly caramelized, slightly crunchy version will likely change their mind.
Serve it hot with Curried Eggplant Parmesan (page 182) and Grilled
Lemon Chicken (page 221) or cold, dipped in hummus, for an
appetizer.

> 1 large head cauliflower, cut into florets
>
> ¼ cup extra-virgin olive oil
>
> 1 tablespoon ground cumin
>
> 1½ teaspoons garlic powder
>
> ½ teaspoon sea salt
>
> 3 tablespoons freshly squeezed lemon juice

Preheat the oven to 425°F.

In a large bowl, toss the cauliflower florets with the oil. Sprinkle
with the cumin, garlic powder, and salt and toss to combine. Spread
the cauliflower evenly on a baking sheet and drizzle with 2 tablespoons
of the lemon juice.

Roast for 15 minutes, gently toss, and roast for another 10 minutes,
or until the cauliflower is golden brown and tender. Drizzle on the
remaining 1 tablespoon lemon juice.

Rainbow Salad

Prep time: 15 minutes
Serves 4 to 6

Adding a least one little surprise ingredient can make any salad special. This can be anything from a sprinkling of your favorite crumbly cheese, avocado slices, toasted nuts, dried fruit, or in this case, some sweet and crunchy sesame sticks. Crunchy chow mein noodles are a nice substitution if you can't find sesame sticks in the grocery store.

3 cups chopped romaine lettuce

3 cups baby spinach

1 cucumber, sliced

2 carrots, peeled and cut into matchsticks

3 radishes, thinly sliced

½ cup frozen shelled edamame, thawed

¼ cup chopped fresh mint

¼ cup chopped fresh cilantro

1 cup honey sesame sticks

Dressing

¼ cup orange juice

Juice of ½ lime

2 tablespoons tahini

1 tablespoon honey

2 tablespoons toasted sesame oil

2 tablespoons extra-virgin olive oil

In a large bowl, combine the romaine, spinach, cucumber, carrots, radishes, and edamame. Top with the mint, cilantro, and sesame sticks. In a small bowl, whisk together the orange juice, lime juice, tahini, and honey. Slowly whisk in the sesame oil and olive oil. Pour the dressing over the salad and lightly toss to combine.

Orzo and Zucchini with Garlic

Prep time: 10 minutes
Cook time: 15 minutes
Serves 4 to 5

Loaded with delicate zucchini and slightly sweet tomatoes, this simple dish is a perfect way to satisfy a pasta craving without going overboard. Kids will devour it. It's a great side for any protein, and it tastes delicious with chopped spinach the next day for lunch.

1½ cups orzo (whole wheat if possible)

3 tablespoons extra-virgin olive oil

2 garlic cloves, chopped

1 large zucchini, grated

1½ cups halved cherry tomatoes

½ teaspoon sea salt

½ teaspoon ground black pepper

¼ cup chopped fresh parsley

Bring a medium pot of water to a boil over high heat. Add the orzo and cook for 5 to 7 minutes, or until the pasta is mostly cooked but still has a slight bite (al dente). Drain and set aside.

Heat 1 tablespoon of the oil in a medium sauté pan over medium-high heat. Add the garlic and sauté for 30 seconds. Add the grated zucchini and cook for 3 to 5 minutes, or until slightly tender.

Add the tomatoes and cook for 2 to 3 minutes, until the tomatoes are slightly cooked but still firm. Season with the salt and pepper, and remove the pan from the heat. Add the cooked orzo and remaining 2 tablespoons oil to the pan. Toss until it's well incorporated. Top with the parsley.

Asian Slaw

Prep time: 15 minutes
Cook time: 8 minutes
Serves 6

This salad is a crowd pleaser and can hold its own as a light lunch or dinner. It can also keep for days and be served as leftovers. Try pairing it with Ahi Tuna Medallions (page 223) or Pistachio-Crusted Chicken (page 215) for a heartier meal.

- 4 ounces whole-wheat spaghetti
- 2 large carrots, peeled and shaved into ribbons with a vegetable peeler
- 2 cups shredded purple cabbage
- 1 large red pepper, thinly sliced
- 1½ cups small broccoli florets
- 3 scallions, finely chopped

Dressing

- ¼ cup orange juice
- ¼ cup natural peanut butter
- 3 tablespoons low-sodium soy sauce or tamari
- Juice of 1 lime

2 tablespoons honey

2 tablespoons extra-virgin olive oil

½ teaspoon red chili paste (optional)

¼ cup chopped fresh cilantro

Bring a medium pot of water to a boil over high heat. Add the spaghetti and cook for 8 minutes, or until the pasta is mostly cooked but still has a slight bite (al dente). Drain and rinse under cold water.

In a large bowl, combine the spaghetti, carrots, cabbage, red pepper, broccoli, and scallions. Toss to combine.

In a small bowl, whisk together all the dressing ingredients. Pour the dressing over the salad and gently toss. Top with the cilantro.

Sautéed Broccolini with Lemony Brazil Nuts

Prep time: 10 minutes
Cook time: 10 minutes
Serves 4

Broccolini is similar to broccoli, but it has smaller florets and a longer, thinner stem. It is also slightly sweeter than broccoli, and the entire vegetable is edible, including the leaves. This dish is simple but loaded with flavor. It can be eaten on its own as a snack or as an accompaniment to any meat or vegetarian meal. Brazil nuts add a buttery flavor to this dish, but almost any nut could be used.

5 Brazil nuts, finely chopped

2 tablespoons grated lemon zest

¼ teaspoon sea salt

1½ tablespoons extra-virgin olive oil

1 pound broccolini, bottoms trimmed

¼ cup water

2 tablespoons low-sodium soy sauce or tamari

In a large sauté pan, lightly toast the Brazil nuts over medium heat for 2 to 4 minutes, or until they're light golden and fragrant. Transfer to a shallow bowl and gently mix in the lemon zest and salt while the nuts are still warm.

Heat the oil in the same pan over medium-high heat. Add the broccolini and sauté for 3 to 4 minutes. Add the water and soy sauce, then cover to steam. Cook for 4 to 6 minutes, or until the broccolini is fork tender and bright green. Transfer to a plate and top with the lemony Brazil nuts.

Roasted Maple Brussels Sprouts

Prep time: 15 minutes
Cook time: 25 minutes
Serves 4

Brussels sprouts are grown in abundance and can be found throughout much of the year. This recipe is simple to make and a pleaser for even the pickiest eater.

1 pound brussels sprouts

¼ cup pure maple syrup

2 tablespoons extra-virgin olive oil

¼ teaspoon sea salt

¼ teaspoon ground black pepper

Preheat the oven to 400°F. Line a rimmed baking sheet with aluminum foil.

Trim the ends of the brussels sprouts. Cut them in half and rinse them under cold water. Pat dry with a towel and transfer them to the baking sheet. Drizzle on the maple syrup and oil, mix to coat, then season with the salt and pepper. Place the baking sheet on the middle rack of the oven and roast for 15 minutes. Gently shake the pan or stir lightly with a spoon. Roast for another 10 minutes, or until the brussels sprouts are golden brown and tender.

CHAPTER 12

Beans and Legumes

Beans and legumes are high in protein, fiber, minerals, and anti-oxidants and are known to help prevent disease, too. They're easy to find in most parts of the world year-round. Whether dry or canned, they keep well, so stock your pantry! Beans can be transformed into a burger, salad base, breakfast side, refried bean leftover, or grain buddy for quick and delicious meals.

If you can, choose dried beans or legumes rather than canned. Dried beans are more cost-effective, have no sodium or preservatives, are tastier, are environmentally friendly, come in more varieties, and allow for greater control in cooking. And though canned beans do save time, a little planning makes working with dried beans not much different. Dried beans (except for most lentils) need to be soaked for a few hours or overnight and then drained before cooking. Check the package instructions or do a quick Internet search for specific instructions regarding the type of legume you are planning to prepare so you will know how much advance prep time is necessary.

Cool Lentil Salad

Prep time: 15 minutes
Cook time: 20 minutes
Serves 4

Lentils are a staple in many parts of the world. With their high protein and fiber content, and healthy supply of vitamins and minerals, they are definitely a superfood. Cold lentil salads are a delicious and convenient way to get your legumes. This dish can be made ahead of time and enjoyed throughout the week. Add any other veggies you may have on hand.

Dressing

> 3 tablespoons freshly squeezed orange juice
>
> 1 tablespoon red wine vinegar
>
> 1 tablespoon grated orange zest
>
> ¼ cup extra-virgin olive oil

Lentils

> 1 cup green lentils
>
> 4 cups water or vegetable broth

Vegetables

> 1 tablespoon extra-virgin olive oil
>
> 1 small zucchini, diced
>
> 1 orange bell pepper, seeded and chopped
>
> ¼ cup chopped fresh dill
>
> ⅓ cup crumbled light feta cheese
>
> ¼ teaspoon sea salt
>
> ¼ teaspoon ground black pepper

In a small bowl, whisk together the orange juice, vinegar, and orange zest. Slowly whisk in the oil.

Sort through the lentils to remove any pebbles or discolored lentils. Rinse the lentils thoroughly under cold water. In a medium pot, bring the lentils and water to a boil over high heat. Reduce the heat and simmer, uncovered, for 15 to 20 minutes, or until the lentils are cooked through and tender with a slight bite. Drain and rinse with cold water.

Heat the oil in a medium sauté pan over medium-high heat. Add the zucchini and bell pepper and sauté for 2 to 3 minutes, or until slightly cooked but still a little crunchy. Transfer to a medium bowl. Add the lentils, dill, feta, salt, and pepper. Pour the dressing over the salad and mix. It's okay if the veggies are still warm; it'll help harmonize the flavors.

Roasted Chickpeas with Creamy Feta Dressing

Prep time: 10 minutes
Cook time: 20 minutes
Serves: 6

Chickpeas are high in protein and fiber, and they offer a healthy dose of minerals. This superfood is also versatile enough to be prepared in many ways and in many forms. Here the chickpeas are roasted for a quick and comforting vegetarian meal — and delicious leftovers the following day.

1 tablespoon dried parsley

1 teaspoon ground cumin

½ teaspoon ground coriander

½ teaspoon smoked paprika

½ teaspoon garlic salt

1½ cups cooked chickpeas *or* 1 (15-ounce) can chickpeas, rinsed and drained

3 tablespoons extra-virgin olive oil

4 Roma tomatoes, diced

1 small red onion, diced

¼ teaspoon sea salt

Dressing

⅓ cup low-fat plain Greek yogurt

¼ cup crumbled light feta cheese

1 tablespoon tahini

1 tablespoon freshly squeezed lemon juice

¼ teaspoon sea salt

Preheat the oven to 400°F. Line two rimmed baking sheets with aluminum foil.

In a medium bowl, combine the dried parsley, cumin, coriander, smoked paprika, and garlic salt. Add the chickpeas and 1 tablespoon of the olive oil and toss until well combined. Transfer to one of the baking sheets and spread the chickpeas out so they are not crowded together.

In a medium bowl, combine the tomatoes, onion, remaining 2 tablespoons olive oil, and salt. Transfer to the other baking sheet. Roast the chickpeas and vegetables for 20 minutes.

In a small bowl, whisk together all the dressing ingredients. Transfer the roasted chickpeas and vegetables to a serving dish and gently toss them together. Top with the yogurt-feta dressing.

Black Bean and Corn Salad

Prep time: 5 minutes
Serves 4

This salad is delicious, satisfying, and incredibly simple to make. It's also full of fiber, vitamin C, protein, and healthy carbohydrates. It makes a fantastic lunch on its own or a perfect accompaniment to sandwiches, grilled chicken, and fish, so make a big batch of it to have all week long. It is also an easy dish to whip up for a party or cookout. Top with avocado slices for even more nutrients.

> 1½ cups cooked black beans or 1 (15-ounce) can black beans, rinsed and drained
>
> 1 cup fresh or thawed frozen corn
>
> 1 red bell pepper, seeded and chopped

Dressing

> ¼ cup extra-virgin olive oil
>
> 2 tablespoons red wine vinegar
>
> ¼ teaspoon sea salt
>
> ¼ teaspoon ground black pepper

In a large bowl, combine the black beans, corn, and red pepper. In a small bowl, whisk together all the dressing ingredients. Pour over the salad and toss to combine.

Black Bean and Brown Rice Burgers

Prep time: 20 minutes, plus 30 minutes to chill
Cook time: 15 minutes
Serves 8

Veggie burgers are a great way to use up leftover ingredients. All you need are bits and ends of vegetables along with a starchy bean and grain. These black bean burgers are a win for meat eaters and vegetarians alike.

- 1½ cups cooked black beans *or* 1 (15-ounce) can black beans, rinsed and drained
- ½ cup canned diced green chiles, drained
- 1 small yellow onion, finely chopped
- 1 large carrot, peeled and grated
- 1 cup cooked brown rice or other grain
- ⅓ cup whole-wheat breadcrumbs
- 1 large egg, beaten
- ¼ cup chopped fresh cilantro
- 1 garlic clove, chopped
- 1 teaspoon ground cumin
- 1 teaspoon garlic salt
- ¼ teaspoon ground ancho or chipotle chile
- 4 tablespoons extra-virgin olive oil, plus more if needed
- 8 tablespoons orange marmalade
- 5 Roma tomatoes, sliced
- 8 whole-wheat buns, for serving (optional)

Using a potato masher or food processor, mash or pulse the black beans until there are no whole beans intact, but do not puree.

In a large bowl, combine the mashed beans, green chiles, onion, carrot, and rice. Stir in the breadcrumbs and egg. Add the cilantro, garlic, cumin, garlic salt, and ground chile. Stir until well incorporated.

Using a ⅓-cup measure, scoop out the mixture and form into eight patties. Place on a plate, cover, and freeze for 30 minutes or refrigerate for 2 hours. The colder the patties are, the better they'll hold their shape when cooking.

Heat 2 tablespoons of the oil in a large sauté pan over medium-high heat. Add four patties and cook for 3 to 5 minutes per side, or until they have a light golden crust. Transfer to a plate. Add the remaining 2 tablespoons oil and cook the remaining four patties in the same manner, adding more oil to the pan if it gets dry.

Spread 1 tablespoon of marmalade on each burger, top with tomato slices, and serve on a bun, if desired.

Vegan Split Pea Soup

Prep time: 20 minutes
Cook time: 1 hour 10 minutes
Serves 8

The traditional version of split pea soup uses a ham bone, but this meatless version is just as tasty. It's also loaded with healthy carbohydrates and lean, plant-based protein. Make a big pot and eat it throughout the week. The soup can hold its own as a meal or is great with a sandwich or a slice of quality whole-grain bread.

1 ounce dried mushrooms

2 tablespoons extra-virgin olive oil

1 cup diced carrot

1 cup diced celery

1 large yellow onion, diced

½ teaspoon sea salt

¼ teaspoon ground black pepper

2 tablespoons grainy mustard

2 cups split peas, rinsed

2 quarts low-sodium vegetable broth

1 bay leaf

Put the dried mushrooms in a small bowl and cover with tepid water. Soak for 15 minutes to rehydrate, then drain the mushrooms and rinse well. Roughly chop the mushrooms.

Heat the oil in a large pot over medium heat. Add the carrot, celery, onion, salt, and pepper. Sauté for 5 to 7 minutes, or until the onion is translucent. Add the mushrooms and mustard and sauté for 2 minutes. Add the split peas, broth, and bay leaf. Raise the heat to medium-high and bring to a boil. Reduce the heat to medium and simmer for 45 to 60 minutes, or until the peas are tender. Remove the bay leaf before serving.

Herbed Tomato and Lentil Soup

Prep time: 15 minutes
Cook time: 40 minutes
Serves 8

Tomato soup is one of the most familiar and comforting meals out there, and this version is packed with tomato flavor and fresh herbs, plus an extra protein boost from lentils. You can add a handful of spinach or other greens or a drizzle of balsamic vinegar reduction for added flavor.

2 tablespoons extra-virgin olive oil

1 yellow onion, diced

2 tablespoons chopped fresh rosemary

1 tablespoon chopped fresh thyme

3 tablespoons tomato paste

¼ cup dry white wine

2 (15-ounce) cans diced tomatoes, undrained

1 cup green lentils, rinsed

2 quarts low-sodium vegetable broth

½ teaspoon sea salt

¼ teaspoon ground black pepper

¼ cup chopped fresh parsley

¼ cup chopped fresh basil

Heat the oil in a large pot over medium-high heat. Add the onion, rosemary, and thyme and sauté for 2 minutes, or until the onion is translucent. Add the tomato paste and sauté for 1½ minutes. Deglaze the pan with the wine. Add the diced tomatoes with their juice, lentils, and broth. Bring to a boil, reduce the heat to medium, and simmer for 30 to 40 minutes, or until the lentils are tender. Season with the salt and pepper, then top with the parsley and basil.

Black-Eyed Pea Summer Salad

Prep time: 15 minutes
Cook time: 25 minutes
Serves 4 to 5

If you've never tried black-eyed peas, I highly recommend that you do so now! This light, refreshing summer salad is perfect on its own as a complete meal for lunch. You can also jazz it up by adding your favorite leafy green or protein. This salad is a crowd pleaser and travels well, so bring it to your next cookout or potluck.

   5 cups water

   ½ cup pearl barley, rinsed

   1½ cups cooked black-eyed peas *or* 1 (15-ounce) can black-eyed peas, rinsed and drained

   1 cup fresh or thawed frozen corn

   1 cucumber, peeled and diced

   2 tablespoons minced red onion

   ¼ cup chopped fresh dill

   ¼ cup fresh basil chiffonade (thin ribbons)

Dressing

   ¼ cup extra-virgin olive oil

   3 tablespoons apple cider vinegar

   ¼ teaspoon sea salt

   ¼ teaspoon ground black pepper

Bring the water to a boil in a medium pot over medium-high heat. Add the barley, reduce the heat to a simmer, and cook for 20 to 25 minutes, or until tender and chewy. Drain and set aside.

In a large bowl, combine the black-eyed peas, corn, cucumber, onion, dill, and basil. Stir in the barley. In a small bowl, whisk together the oil and vinegar. Pour the dressing over the salad and toss to combine. Season with the salt and pepper.

Refried Black and Pinto Beans

Prep time: 10 minutes
Cook time: 10 minutes
Serves 6

Refried beans are both tasty and popular, and this delicious version is lighter in fat than the traditional dish but still packed with flavor. Enjoy these beans with simple brown rice or in a tortilla wrap with sautéed onions and bell peppers. They are also great as a hearty dip topped with avocado and diced tomatoes.

⅓ cup extra-virgin olive oil

1½ cups cooked black beans plus ½ cup cooking liquid or water *or* 1 (15-ounce) can black beans, undrained

1½ cups cooked pinto beans plus ½ cup cooking liquid or water *or* 1 (15-ounce can) pinto beans, undrained

½ tablespoon garlic powder

½ tablespoon onion powder

1 teaspoon ground cumin

½ teaspoon sea salt

½ teaspoon paprika

¼ teaspoon chili powder

Heat the oil in a medium sauté pan over medium-high heat. Add the beans and liquid and bring to a heavy simmer. Add the garlic powder, onion powder, cumin, salt, paprika, and chili powder. Reduce to a light simmer and cook for 10 minutes.

Remove the pan from the heat. Using a potato masher, break up the beans until they're smooth or leave them slightly chunky, as desired.

Quinoa-Chickpea Patties

Prep time: 20 minutes, plus 30 minutes to chill
Cook time: 30 minutes
Serves 6

These veggie patties are so hearty and chock-full of protein and fiber that even the most voracious meat lover will be satisfied. We like to serve these over tender Bibb lettuce topped with tomato and avocado slices, but you could also go the traditional route with a whole-wheat bun. A dollop of tzatziki or pesto is a great option as a condiment.

½ cup quinoa, rinsed

1 cup water

1½ cups cooked chickpeas plus ¼ cup cooking liquid or water *or* 1 (15-ounce) can chickpeas, reserve ¼ cup liquid

1 carrot, peeled and grated

2 garlic cloves, minced

1 large egg, beaten

⅓ cup whole-wheat breadcrumbs

¼ cup chickpea flour or whole-wheat flour

¼ cup chopped fresh parsley

1 tablespoon ground cumin

½ teaspoon smoked paprika

½ teaspoon sea salt

4 tablespoons extra-virgin olive oil, plus more if needed

1 head Bibb lettuce, separated into leaves

2 avocados, peeled, pitted, and thinly sliced

4 Roma tomatoes, thinly sliced

In a small pot, bring the quinoa and water to a boil over medium-high heat. Reduce the heat to low, cover, and cook for 15 to 20 minutes, or until light and fluffy.

Pour the chickpeas and liquid into a food processor and pulse to break up the chickpeas until they're mostly mashed—a little chunky is okay. (If you do not have a food processor, a potato masher will do the trick.) Transfer to a large bowl and add the quinoa, carrot, garlic, egg, breadcrumbs, flour, parsley, cumin, paprika, and salt. Mix until well combined. The mixture should be slightly sticky; add a little water if it's too dry.

Using a ⅓-cup measure, scoop out the mixture and form into six patties. Place on a plate, cover, and freeze for 30 minutes or refrigerate for 2 hours. The colder the patties are, the better they'll hold their shape when cooking.

Heat 2 tablespoons of the oil in a large sauté pan over medium-high heat. Add three patties and cook for 3 to 5 minutes per side, or until a light golden crust appears. Transfer to a plate. Add the remaining 2 tablespoons oil and cook the remaining three patties in the same manner, adding more oil to the pan if it gets dry. Place each patty on a few lettuce leaves and top with avocado and tomato slices.

Huevos Rancheros with Blistered Tomatoes

Prep time: 20 minutes
Cook time: 15 minutes
Serves 4

Huevos rancheros translates to "ranch eggs" in Spanish and is typically served with crispy corn tortillas and a fried egg. This version is made with black beans and blistered sweet cherry tomatoes for a hearty meal any time of day. Top with avocado slices or a dollop of low-fat yogurt.

    3 tablespoons extra-virgin olive oil

    2 tablespoons honey

    ¼ teaspoon chili powder

    ¼ teaspoon sea salt

    1 pound cherry tomatoes

    1½ cups cooked black beans plus ½ cup cooking liquid or water
      or 1 (15-ounce) can black beans, undrained

    1 teaspoon garlic powder

    ½ teaspoon ground cumin

    8 corn tortillas

    1 tablespoon extra-virgin olive oil

    4 large eggs

In a medium bowl, whisk together the olive oil, honey, chili powder, and salt. Add the tomatoes and toss until they're lightly coated. Heat a large sauté pan over high heat. Add the tomatoes and let them sit for 2 minutes, or until slightly charred on the bottom. Stir the tomatoes and let them blister for another 2 to 3 minutes. Remove from the heat.

In a medium pot, combine the beans and liquid, garlic powder, and cumin. Simmer over medium-high heat for 5 minutes. Remove from the heat.

On a microwave-safe plate, microwave the corn tortillas in batches on high for 2 to 4 minutes, or until soft.

Heat the oil in a large sauté pan over medium heat. Crack the eggs into the pan, taking care not to break the yolks. Cook the eggs for 2 to 4 minutes, or until the whites are set. Gently flip, making sure not to break the yolks. Cook for another minute for over-easy, or until your preferred doneness.

To assemble, place two corn tortillas on each plate. Top with one-quarter of the black beans, a fried egg, and one-quarter of the tomatoes.

CHAPTER 13

Seafood and Poultry

Seafood and poultry are terrific for brain health, and they're also one of the healthiest sources of protein per serving. One 4-ounce serving provides anywhere from 25 to 35 grams of protein. Here are a few ways to prepare your seafood and poultry:

- *Grilled:* This is a favorite cooking method because of the slightly smoky taste it imparts. Grilling can dry out fish and poultry, so it is a good idea to use a marinade. The marinade also helps reduce the carcinogenic effect of grilling by creating a protective layer around the meat. The best types of fish for the grill are thick, meaty cuts, such as salmon, tuna, mahi-mahi, and swordfish.

- *Baked or Roasted:* Cooking fish or poultry in the oven is an ideal method. The slow heat penetration ensures even cooking throughout the protein without drying it out. A marinade, dry rub, or simply salt and pepper can be used to add flavor.

- *Sautéed:* Sautéing your protein is quick, easy, and satisfying. You can get a nice sear or crust on the outside and a delicate texture on the inside. You can use marinades or dry rubs. Be sure to go light on oil when you're sautéing.

- *Steamed/Poached:* Steaming or poaching fish or poultry is a great way to preserve flavor and lock in moisture. It is a lighter cooking method, since typically no fat is used, and lots of flavor can be added by using different aromatics and liquids. This is the best way to prepare fish so that it doesn't dry out. It is a bit harder to cook poultry this way, because it can cook unevenly and get rubbery.

Baked Shrimp and Scallops

Prep time: 15 minutes
Cook time: 15 minutes
Serves 3 to 4

Baking shrimp and scallops is quick and easy but yields elegant results. This dish pairs beautifully with Fresh and Light Garlicky Linguine (page 158) or Quinoa and Kale with Toasted Pine Nuts (page 157). For a delicious light summer meal, serve it with a seasonal fresh salad.

Juice of 1 lemon

¼ cup dry white wine

3 tablespoons extra-virgin olive oil

2 garlic cloves, minced

¼ cup chopped fresh parsley

8 large shrimp, peeled and deveined

8 large scallops, side muscles removed

Preheat the oven to 350°F. Line two rimmed baking sheets with aluminum foil.

In a large bowl, whisk together the lemon juice, white wine, olive oil, garlic, and parsley. Add the shrimp and scallops and toss so they're well coated. Using tongs, transfer the shrimp to one baking sheet and the scallops to the other. Bake the shrimp for 8 minutes, or just until they're pink. Bake the scallops for 12 to 15 minutes, or until they're mostly cooked through and slightly translucent in the center. Combine the shrimp and scallops in a serving bowl and serve hot.

Mediterranean Turkey Burgers

Prep time: 10 minutes
Cook time: 20 minutes
Serves 5

The fresh herbs and hearty sun-dried tomatoes in these turkey burgers make for a vibrant taste in each bite—so much so that you can forgo condiments. Try them topped with tomatoes in a lettuce wrap or on a light whole-wheat bun.

1 pound lean ground turkey

1 large egg, beaten

⅓ cup whole-wheat breadcrumbs

⅓ cup finely chopped oil-packed sun-dried tomatoes

½ cup crumbled light feta cheese

1 tablespoon Dijon mustard

1 teaspoon Worcestershire sauce

¼ cup chopped fresh parsley

2 tablespoons finely chopped fresh dill

1 teaspoon garlic powder

¼ teaspoon sea salt

2 tablespoons extra-virgin olive oil

5 large Bibb lettuce leaves, for serving (optional)

5 whole-wheat buns, for serving (optional)

In a large bowl, gently mix the turkey, egg, and breadcrumbs. Add the sun-dried tomatoes, feta cheese, mustard, Worcestershire sauce, parsley, dill, garlic powder, and salt; mix until everything is well incorporated. Form the mixture into five patties.

Heat 1 tablespoon of the oil in a large sauté pan or grill pan over medium-high heat. Add two patties and cook for 3 to 5 minutes, or until they're a light golden brown on the bottom. Flip them over and reduce the heat to medium-low. Cover the pan and cook the patties for an additional 5 to 7 minutes, or until they're cooked through. Transfer to a plate. Add the remaining 1 tablespoon oil to the pan and cook the remaining three patties in the same manner. Serve in lettuce wraps or buns.

Pistachio-Crusted Chicken

Prep time: 20 minutes
Cook time: 20 minutes
Serves 4

These chicken tenders are tastier and a whole lot healthier than your average fried chicken. Be prepared for your family and friends to devour them—you'll want to make large batches for leftovers. The Dijon supplies a tangy depth, while the chicken stays moist and tender. You can use pecans in place of pistachios and add any fresh herb you want.

1 cup Dijon mustard

3 tablespoons finely chopped fresh rosemary

2 cups panko breadcrumbs (preferably whole-wheat)

½ cup finely chopped pistachios

¼ teaspoon sea salt

¼ teaspoon ground black pepper

8 chicken tenders *or* 1 pound boneless, skinless chicken breasts, cut into 8 tenders

1 tablespoon extra-virgin olive oil

Preheat the oven to 400°F. Line a rimmed baking sheet with aluminum foil and lightly grease or spray the foil with olive oil.

In a shallow dish, mix the Dijon mustard and rosemary. In another shallow dish, combine the panko breadcrumbs, pistachios, salt, and pepper.

Dip the chicken tenders in the Dijon mixture until they're generously coated. Then dredge them in the panko mixture. Place in a single layer on the baking sheet. Lightly drizzle or spray olive oil on top of the tenders.

Bake for 10 minutes, flip the tenders, then bake for an additional 10 minutes.

Spicy Salmon Summer Salad

Prep time: 15 minutes
Cook time: 10 minutes
Serves 4

Salmon and fresh salad is the perfect meal for the mind, as it's light on calories and heavy on brain-healthy ingredients. This duo makes for a great lunch or dinner. We love how the spicy salmon pairs with the sweet maple dressing. Serve with red quinoa for a slightly heartier meal.

- 1 teaspoon paprika
- 1 teaspoon ground cumin
- ½ teaspoon cayenne pepper
- ¼ teaspoon sea salt
- 4 (4-ounce) boneless, skin-on salmon fillets
- 1 tablespoon extra-virgin olive oil

Salad

- 4 cups baby spinach
- 1 head Bibb lettuce, lightly chopped
- 1 cup fresh or thawed frozen corn
- 2 cups halved grape tomatoes

Dressing

- ¼ cup extra-virgin olive oil
- Juice of 1 lime
- 1 tablespoon pure maple syrup

- 2 avocados, peeled, pitted, and sliced
- 2 limes, quartered, for serving

In a small bowl, combine the paprika, cumin, cayenne, and salt. Gently rub the spice mixture onto the flesh side of the salmon fillets. Heat the oil in a large sauté pan over medium heat. Place the fillets, skin-side up, in the pan. Cook for 4 minutes, then flip the fillets. Reduce the heat to low, cover, and cook for another 4 to 6 minutes, or until just cooked through.

In a medium bowl, combine the spinach, lettuce, corn, and tomatoes. In a small bowl, whisk together all the dressing ingredients. Pour the dressing over the salad and toss.

Evenly divide the salad among four plates. Top each with a salmon fillet and a few avocado slices, and serve with the lime wedges on the side.

Pulled Sweet and Tangy Chicken

Prep time: 10 minutes
Cook time: 20 minutes
Serves 4

This is a comforting, no-fuss, kid-friendly meal. The chicken has a delicate balance of sweet, acidic, and rich tomato flavor. It can be served on a bun, in a lettuce wrap, or alongside crunchy coleslaw or some roasted vegetables.

1/3 cup pure maple syrup

1/4 cup tomato paste

1/4 cup rice wine vinegar

1/4 cup low-sodium soy sauce or tamari

1 tablespoon garlic powder

1 tablespoon extra-virgin olive oil

1 pound boneless, skinless chicken breasts

In a medium bowl, whisk together the maple syrup, tomato paste, vinegar, soy sauce, and garlic powder.

In a Dutch oven or heavy pot, heat the oil over medium heat. Add the chicken and the sauce. Using tongs, roll the chicken in the sauce to fully coat it. Cover and cook for 10 minutes, or until the chicken is just cooked through. Transfer each chicken breast, one at a time, to a cutting board and use two forks to gently shred the chicken. Return the shredded chicken to the pot and mix it back into the sauce. Turn the heat to low, cover, and cook for another 10 minutes.

Stuffed Sea Bass with Steamed Vegetables

Prep time: 20 minutes
Cook time: 25 minutes
Serves 4

Sea bass is a delicious, hearty white fish. Cooking vegetables with the fish adds an aromatic depth and flavor. You can serve this as is for a light dinner or pair it with a whole-grain dish like Fresh and Light Garlicky Linguini (page 158). This recipe, loaded with brain-nourishing ingredients, is great for dinner parties, because it can be made ahead of time and popped in the oven when company arrives.

3 cups chopped spinach

2 garlic cloves, minced

1 cup chopped fresh parsley

3 ounces goat cheese

4 (4-ounce) boneless, skinless sea bass fillets

1½ teaspoons chopped fresh rosemary

½ teaspoon sea salt

¼ teaspoon ground black pepper

2 red bell peppers, seeded and diced

1 red onion, diced

1 zucchini, cut into ½-inch rounds

½ cup dry white wine

1 tablespoon extra-virgin olive oil

Preheat the oven to 375°F.

In a small bowl, combine the spinach, garlic, ½ cup of the parsley, and the goat cheese.

Carefully butterfly each fish fillet by slicing it horizontally, leaving about ½ inch still intact at the edge. Spoon a quarter of the spinach mixture into each fillet and lightly press down to close it over the filling. Top each fillet with the chopped rosemary, salt, and pepper.

In a 9-by-11-inch glass baking dish, combine the red peppers, onion, zucchini, remaining ½ cup parsley, white wine, and olive oil. Place the fillets on top of the vegetables, gently pressing them down into the veggies. Cover tightly with aluminum foil and bake for 20 to 25 minutes, or until the fish flakes apart easily.

Salmon with Red Onion and Asparagus

Prep time: 10 minutes
Cook time: 20 minutes
Serves 4

This is the simplest way to prepare a beautiful piece of salmon. There is so much flavor in wild-caught and even farmed salmon that you need only a few ingredients to enjoy this lovely fish.

1 tablespoon extra-virgin olive oil

1 (20-ounce) boneless, skin-on salmon fillet

¼ teaspoon sea salt

¼ teaspoon ground black pepper

1 large lemon, sliced

1 red onion, sliced

1 pound asparagus, trimmed and halved lengthwise if thick

Dressing

¼ cup extra-virgin olive oil

1 tablespoon red wine vinegar

1 tablespoon honey

1½ teaspoons Dijon mustard

Preheat the oven to 375°F. Line a rimmed baking sheet with aluminum foil.

Lightly oil the skin side of the fish and place it in the center of the baking sheet. Season the salmon with the salt and pepper, then place the lemon slices on top, followed by the onion slices. Evenly spread the asparagus on top. Tightly cover the baking sheet with a second piece of foil. Bake for 15 to 20 minutes, or until just cooked through; the cooking time will depend on the thickness of the fillet.

While the fish is baking, in a small bowl, whisk together all the dressing ingredients. Once the fish has cooked, carefully open the foil and transfer the fish and vegetables to a serving plate. Drizzle the dressing over the warm fish just before serving.

Grilled Lemon Chicken

Prep time: 10 minutes, plus 30 minutes to marinate
Cook time: 15 minutes
Serves 4

Grilled chicken is flavorful on its own, but a lemony marinade takes it to a whole new level. This chicken is so tender and versatile, you can pair it with many different dishes. Make a double batch so you can have leftovers for lunch over a big green salad or in a whole-wheat wrap with tzatziki.

⅓ cup extra-virgin olive oil

¼ cup freshly squeezed lemon juice

1 tablespoon dried oregano

1 tablespoon dried minced onion

1 teaspoon garlic powder

½ teaspoon sea salt

½ teaspoon ground black pepper

4 (6-ounce) boneless, skinless chicken breasts

In a shallow bowl, whisk together the olive oil, lemon juice, oregano, minced onion, garlic powder, salt, and pepper. Add the chicken and turn to coat thoroughly. Cover and refrigerate for at least 30 minutes or up to 2 hours.

Heat a grill pan over medium-high heat. Sear each side of the chicken breasts for 2 to 3 minutes, or until dark grill marks appear. Lower the heat, cover, and cook for another 5 to 7 minutes, or until the chicken is cooked through.

Turkey Meatballs

Prep time: 15 minutes
Cook time: 15 minutes
Serves 4

Everyone loves a traditional spaghetti and meatball dish. For a delicious alternative, serve these turkey meatballs over whole-wheat pasta and your favorite tomato sauce.

1 pound lean ground turkey

⅓ cup whole-wheat breadcrumbs

1 large egg, beaten

1 tablespoon Worcestershire sauce or low-sodium soy sauce

1 tablespoon horseradish or Dijon mustard

¼ cup diced yellow onion

½ cup chopped fresh parsley

1 tablespoon dried minced onion

½ teaspoon garlic salt

1 teaspoon dried oregano

Preheat the oven to 375°F. Line a rimmed baking sheet with aluminum foil and lightly grease or spray the foil with olive oil.

Combine all the ingredients in a large bowl and mix thoroughly. Roll the mixture into meatballs the size of golf balls, and place them on the baking sheet.

Bake for 15 minutes, or until cooked through.

Ahi Tuna Medallions

Prep time: 8 minutes, plus 30 minutes to marinate
Cook time: 5 minutes
Serves 4

These tuna medallions will knock your socks off. Ahi tuna alone is so succulent that when it's combined with the fresh acidity of lime and depth of soy sauce, it will really impress. The fish's healthy fats and mega dose of healthy protein will make your brain happy, too! We love this dish paired with Spinach Salad with Peanut Dressing (page 168) or Sautéed Broccolini with Lemony Brazil Nuts (page 191) for a meal that's light on carbohydrates and colorfully decadent.

Marinade

¼ cup extra-virgin olive oil

¼ cup freshly squeezed lime juice

3 tablespoons low-sodium soy sauce or tamari

2 tablespoons honey

2 garlic cloves, chopped

¾ cup chopped fresh cilantro

Grated zest of 1 lime

1 pound ahi tuna steak, cut into 12 (1-inch) pieces

1 lime, quartered, for serving

In a large bowl, whisk together all the marinade ingredients. Add the tuna pieces and stir to coat. Cover and refrigerate for 30 minutes.

Heat a large sauté pan over medium-high heat. Place half of the tuna pieces in the pan. Sear each side for 1 to 1½ minutes, or to the desired doneness. Transfer to a plate and cook the remaining tuna in the same manner. Serve with the lime wedges on the side.

CHAPTER 14

Entertaining

Socializing around food can give you some of your most cherished moments with friends and family. The smells and tastes of various dishes become tied to memories from holidays and special occasions.

If you're hosting a gathering, make sure to ask your guests about their dietary needs and restrictions to make sure everyone enjoys their meal. And when you're deciding on your menu, keep in mind how much time you'll have to prep (including grocery shopping), the type of crowd you are having over (kids, health nuts, football fans, the elderly, and so on), and what the occasion is. It can be helpful to pick a theme (Greek, Mexican, snacks and bites, seated dinner party) and plan your menu from there. Take into account how much time you'll need to cook before *and* after your guests arrive. We find it helpful to make most of our dishes ahead of time and finish off the cooking once the guests arrive so that we can enjoy their company.

If cooking for a large crowd overwhelms you, don't be shy about asking guests to bring a salad, appetizer, or dessert. People love to contribute. If you are going to a potluck, ask the host what you can bring or suggest a dish that you love to make. If your host loves cooking high-fat, rich food, offer to contribute a salad or vegetable dish so you know there will be nutrient-dense, lighter fare to eat. Most important, have fun and take the time to make your food visually appealing and brain-healthy for your guests.

Roasted Salsa Guacamole

Prep time: 10 minutes
Cook time: 45 minutes
Serves 8

This delicious homemade salsa features brain-healthy avocados. Serve with crackers or corn chips and watch your bowl of guac disappear!

1 green bell pepper, seeded and chopped

3 tomatoes, diced

½ yellow onion, diced

1 jalapeño, seeded if desired and minced

⅓ cup red wine vinegar

2 tablespoons extra-virgin olive oil

2 teaspoons garlic powder

¾ teaspoon sea salt

4 avocados

¼ cup roughly chopped fresh cilantro

1 tablespoon freshly squeezed lime juice

Preheat the oven to 425°F.

In a small roasting pan, combine the bell pepper, tomatoes, onion, jalapeño, red wine vinegar, oil, garlic powder, and ¼ teaspoon of the salt and toss to combine. Bake for 45 minutes, gently stirring halfway through. Let cool.

Once the roasted vegetables have cooled, and just before you're ready to serve the guacamole, peel and halve the avocados. Scoop the flesh into a medium bowl and lightly mash it with a fork. Add the cilantro, lime juice, and remaining ½ teaspoon salt and mix well. Add the roasted vegetables to the bowl and mix until they're thoroughly incorporated.

Pesto Chicken and Roasted Red Pepper Sandwiches

Prep time: 10 minutes
Cook time: 25 minutes
Serves 6

These sandwiches are so flavorful and satisfying—they're perfect for a large crowd at a Super Bowl party or any casual get-together. You can easily omit the chicken for a vegetarian version, too.

1 tablespoon extra-virgin olive oil

¼ teaspoon sea salt

¼ teaspoon ground black pepper

2 (6-ounce) boneless, skinless chicken breasts

1 (12- to 18-inch) whole-wheat baguette

1½ cups basil pesto

1 (10-ounce) jar roasted red peppers, drained and roughly chopped

6 ounces smoked light Gouda cheese, sliced

Preheat the oven to 375°F.

Heat the oil in a medium sauté pan over medium-high heat. Evenly salt and pepper both sides of the chicken breasts and add them to the pan. Cook for 6 minutes, or until golden brown on the bottom. Flip the chicken breasts and reduce the heat to low. Cover the pan and cook for an additional 5 to 7 minutes, or until cooked through. Transfer the chicken breasts to a plate and let them stand for 5 minutes. Cut the chicken into ½-inch-thick slices.

Cut the baguette in half. Generously spread pesto on both cut sides. On the bottom half, layer the chicken slices, roasted red peppers, and Gouda. Close the sandwich with the top half. Cut the sandwich in half and wrap each half tightly in aluminum foil.

Bake for 10 minutes, or until the cheese is melted. Unwrap and carefully cut into 2-inch-wide sandwiches.

Sesame Poke Salad

Prep time: 15 minutes
Serves 4

It is important for the flavor and quality of this dish that you purchase sushi-grade tuna from a reputable grocer or fish market. Look for very little webbing—the fish should be bright pink and clean. If you can't find sushi-grade tuna, sushi-grade salmon will do as well. Or opt for a nice piece of spring salmon and sear it on the stovetop instead. For vegans and vegetarians, tofu is a great option, too.

1½ tablespoons low-sodium soy sauce or tamari

1½ tablespoons rice wine vinegar

1 tablespoon freshly squeezed lime juice

2 teaspoons toasted sesame oil

1 tablespoon sesame seeds

12 ounces sushi-grade yellowfin tuna, cut into ½-inch pieces

½ cup frozen shelled edamame, thawed

½ cup diced pineapple

1 carrot, peeled and shaved into ribbons

1 red bell pepper, seeded and thinly sliced

¼ cup shredded or flaked coconut, toasted

In a medium bowl, whisk together the soy sauce, vinegar, lime juice, sesame oil, and sesame seeds. Add the tuna and toss gently.

In a medium bowl, combine the edamame, pineapple, carrot, and red pepper. Spread out the vegetables on a serving platter and top with the tuna and sauce. Sprinkle on the coconut.

Blackberry-Basil Sangria

Prep time: 15 minutes, plus 30 minutes to chill
Cook time: 10 minutes
Serves 6

This sangria combines brain-healthy blackberries with fresh basil for a refreshing, light summer party drink. It is also a beautiful mix of colors for a festive occasion. The blackberry syrup is made using honey instead of sugar for added nutrients and flavor. You can use sparkling wine if you prefer extra bubbles.

4 cups blackberries

1½ cups fresh basil leaves

1 cup water

½ cup honey

1 (750-ml) bottle dry white wine

1 cup sparkling water

2 limes, cut into ¼-inch rounds

2 cups ice

In a medium saucepan, combine 3 cups of the blackberries, 1 cup of the basil leaves, the water, and honey. Bring to a boil over medium heat and simmer for 10 minutes. Let cool and strain the syrup through a fine-mesh sieve into a glass measuring cup. You should have roughly 1 cup of syrup.

In a serving pitcher, combine the blackberry syrup, wine, and sparkling water. Stir gently. Add the lime slices, remaining ½ cup basil leaves, remaining 1 cup blackberries, and ice. Chill in the refrigerator for at least 30 minutes or up to 4 hours.

Balsamic Pasta Salad with Roasted Asparagus

Prep time: 15 minutes
Cook time: 15 minutes
Serves 8

Pasta salad is a staple at many casual and semi-casual get-togethers because it's a popular dish for all ages and easy to transport. This version has roasted balsamic vegetables, which make it a delicious and healthy alternative to the traditional mayonnaise-based pasta salad. We call for rotini, but you could swap it out for any short variety of whole-grain pasta.

1 pound asparagus, trimmed and cut into 2-inch pieces

1 pint cherry tomatoes, halved

¼ cup plus 2 tablespoons balsamic vinegar

1 teaspoon chopped fresh rosemary

½ teaspoon sea salt

1 pound whole-wheat rotini pasta

¼ cup extra-virgin olive oil

⅓ cup chopped raw walnuts

¼ cup crumbled goat cheese

Preheat the oven to 400°F. Line a rimmed baking sheet with aluminum foil.

In a medium bowl, combine the asparagus pieces, tomatoes, ¼ cup of the balsamic vinegar, rosemary, and salt. Toss and transfer to the baking sheet. Roast for 15 minutes, or until the asparagus is bright green and slightly tender.

Meanwhile, bring a large pot of water to a boil over high heat. Add the rotini and cook for 8 to 10 minutes, or until the pasta is mostly cooked but still has a slight bite (al dente). Drain and rinse under cold water.

In a large bowl, combine the rotini and roasted asparagus and tomatoes. Add the oil and remaining 2 tablespoons balsamic vinegar and toss to coat. Top with the walnuts and goat cheese.

The Best Turkey Sliders

Prep time: 10 minutes, plus 30 minutes to chill
Cook time: 10 minutes
Serves 4

These Asian-seasoned turkey burgers are going to be your new favorite! Packed with flavor and easy to make, they are great for a cookout or lunch party for all ages.

1 pound lean ground turkey

1 large egg, lightly beaten

3 tablespoons low-sodium soy sauce or tamari

2 tablespoons honey

⅓ cup whole-wheat breadcrumbs

⅓ cup chopped fresh cilantro

2 scallions, finely chopped

1 garlic clove, minced

1 tablespoon grated fresh ginger

2 tablespoons extra-virgin olive oil

Tangy Sauce

3 tablespoons ketchup

1 tablespoon Dijon mustard

1½ teaspoons low-sodium soy sauce or tamari

8 whole-wheat slider buns, for serving

In a medium bowl, combine the ground turkey, egg, soy sauce, honey, breadcrumbs, cilantro, scallions, garlic, and ginger and mix until everything is well incorporated. Form into eight small patties and place on a plate. Cover and refrigerate for 30 minutes.

Heat 1 tablespoon of the oil in a large sauté pan over medium-high heat. Add four patties and cook for 2 to 4 minutes per side, or until they're cooked through and golden brown. Transfer to a plate. Add the remaining 1 tablespoon oil to the pan and cook the remaining four patties in the same manner.

In a small bowl, whisk together all the sauce ingredients. Spread the sauce on the burgers and serve on the buns.

Portobello Veggie Stackers

Prep time: 20 minutes
Cook time: 22 minutes
Serves 6

Serve these flavorful portobello veggie stackers for a lunch party with vegetarian guests. You can easily skip the cheese for a vegan option. They're also hearty enough to eat without sides. Try cremini mushrooms for a smaller serving size or an appetizer.

1 large red bell pepper, seeded and cut into 12 squares

1 zucchini, cut into 12 (¼-inch-thick) slices

1 tablespoon plus 1 teaspoon extra-virgin olive oil

¼ teaspoon sea salt

¼ teaspoon ground black pepper

6 portobello mushrooms, stems removed

Pesto

1 cup fresh basil leaves

½ cup raw almonds or pine nuts

⅓ cup water

¼ cup extra-virgin olive oil

¼ teaspoon sea salt

¼ teaspoon ground black pepper

6 tablespoons minced oil-packed sun-dried tomatoes

¾ cup Parmesan cheese shavings

12 small basil leaves, for garnish

Preheat the oven to 400°F. Line two rimmed baking sheets with aluminum foil.

Place the red peppers and zucchini on one of the baking sheets. Add 1 tablespoon of the oil and the salt and pepper and toss to combine. Spread out in a single layer and roast for 20 minutes, stirring halfway through.

While the vegetables are roasting, heat the remaining 1 teaspoon oil in a medium sauté pan over medium-high heat. Add the mushroom caps and cook for 3 to 5 minutes per side, or until golden brown.

In a food processor, combine all the pesto ingredients and pulse until the mixture is smooth.

When the peppers and zucchini are done, set the oven to broil.

Place the mushroom caps, gill-side up, on the other baking sheet. Layer each mushroom cap with 1 tablespoon of sun-dried tomatoes, 1 tablespoon of cheese shavings, two pieces of red bell pepper side by side, 1 tablespoon of pesto, and two zucchini slices side by side. Top with an additional 1 tablespoon each of pesto and cheese shavings.

Broil for 2 minutes, or until the cheese is bubbly. Garnish each stack with 2 basil leaves.

Heirloom Tomato Salad

Prep time: 10 minutes
Cook time: 2 minutes
Serves 4

Salads are a delicious way to sneak in several servings of vegetables. This salad is beautifully presented and filled with flavor. It pairs well with fish or chicken and is great for leftovers.

1½ lemons

3 cups shredded spinach

2 or 3 large heirloom or vine-ripe tomatoes, sliced

⅔ cup sliced Kalamata olives

¼ cup crumbled light feta cheese

1 large cucumber, sliced

1½ teaspoons dried oregano

¼ cup chopped fresh dill

2 tablespoons extra-virgin olive oil

½ cup cooked or canned chickpeas

¼ teaspoon ground black pepper

Slice one of the lemons into 4 or 5 rounds. Put the lemon slices in a medium sauté pan over medium-high heat (no oil is needed). Brown each side for 1 minute. Set aside.

On a large plate or serving platter, evenly distribute the spinach, then top with the tomatoes, olives, and feta cheese. Decoratively arrange the cucumbers around the edge of the salad, making a border. Evenly sprinkle the oregano and dill over the salad. Drizzle with the oil. Top with the chickpeas and pepper. Squeeze the juice from the remaining ½ lemon over the salad and arrange the cooked lemon rounds on top — these can be eaten or used as garnish.

Sautéed Kale and Mushroom Canapés

Prep time: 10 minutes
Cook time: 8 minutes
Serves 8

These canapés are easy to make and full of brain-healthy antioxidants. The simple combination of kale and mushrooms, with just a touch of garlic, makes the perfect light vegetarian appetizer for a party.

1 (12- to 18-inch) whole-wheat baguette, cut on the bias into
 ½-inch-thick slices

3 tablespoons extra-virgin olive oil

1 bunch kale, stems removed and leaves chopped

1 garlic clove, chopped

3 portobello mushrooms, stemmed and thinly sliced

¼ teaspoon sea salt

¼ teaspoon ground black pepper

Preheat the oven to 375°F. Line a rimmed baking sheet with aluminum foil.

Place the baguette slices on the baking sheet. Drizzle 1 tablespoon of the oil evenly over the slices. Bake for 5 to 7 minutes, or until lightly toasted.

Meanwhile, heat the remaining 2 tablespoons oil in a medium sauté pan over medium heat. Sauté the kale for 5 minutes. Add the garlic and sauté for 1 minute. Transfer the kale to a plate. Add the mushrooms to the pan. Cook for 2 minutes on each side, or until golden brown.

On each baguette slice, layer about 1 spoonful of kale and 2 mushroom slices. Sprinkle with the salt and pepper.

Greek Seven-Layer Dip

Prep time: 15 minutes
Cook time: 10 minutes
Serves 8

Looking for a quick, colorful, easy, and delicious appetizer to whip up for a casual get-together or to bring to a party? This creamy, crunchy, savory dip is loaded with veggies. Serve with cut-up veggies, pita chips, or crackers.

2 cups hummus

1 green bell pepper, seeded and chopped

1 cup cherry tomatoes, halved

⅔ cup chopped Kalamata olives

2 tablespoons finely chopped red onion

1 cup diced cucumber

⅓ cup crumbled light feta cheese

2 tablespoons chopped fresh dill

1 tablespoon extra-virgin olive oil

1 teaspoon freshly squeezed lemon juice

On a large plate or serving platter, layer the hummus, green pepper, tomatoes, olives, red onion, cucumber, feta cheese, and dill. Drizzle with the oil and lemon juice.

CHAPTER 15

Snacks and Desserts

When you're in the mood for a snack, use the opportunity to nibble on nuts, fruit, or foods from the food groups you're low on for the day. Snacking on potato chips or other junk foods that carry a low nutrient density will do little to fill you up and will cause harm to your waistline and health. Aim for snacks that combine complex carbohydrates with lean protein to balance blood sugar and to satisfy. Most important, be prepared for a snack attack by knowing when your body will be hungry.

And when you have a craving for dessert, remember that more and more research is pointing to how detrimental sugar is to our health. We are consuming more than ever before, because it is being added to cereals, breads, sauces, drinks, and just about every processed food. To greatly reduce your intake, try limiting sugary drinks and sodas, eliminating processed packaged desserts like cookies, muffins, and pastries, and making your own desserts and snacks. It is important to note that portion control is key to eating dessert—less sugar does not mean you can eat more at one sitting.

Lemon-Roasted Hummus

Prep time: 10 minutes
Cook time: 10 minutes
Serves 4

Hummus really can do it all: Use it as a dip for vegetables and crackers, as a sauce for chicken, as a salad dressing when thinned out, in place of cheese or mayonnaise on a sandwich, or as a binder for breading vegetables and meats. If you are up for making your own, it is super easy and economical. For extra smooth hummus, remove the skins from the chickpeas before pureeing.

- 1½ cups cooked chickpeas *or* 1 (15-ounce) can chickpeas, rinsed and drained
- 2 tablespoons extra-virgin olive oil
- 3 tablespoons freshly squeezed lemon juice
- 1 tablespoon honey
- Grated zest of 1 lemon
- ½ teaspoon sea salt
- ¼ teaspoon ground cardamom
- ⅛ teaspoon ground nutmeg
- ⅓ cup water
- 2 tablespoons tahini

Preheat the oven to 400°F. Line a rimmed baking sheet with aluminum foil.

Combine the chickpeas, oil, lemon juice, honey, lemon zest, salt, cardamom, and nutmeg on the baking sheet and toss to coat well. Spread out the chickpeas on the sheet and bake for 10 minutes. Let cool.

In a blender or food processor, combine the roasted chickpeas, water, and tahini. Blend on high until smooth and creamy.

Kale Chips

Prep time: 10 minutes
Cook time: 15 minutes
Serves 4

These crunchy chips are so good that they'll disappear from your serving plate before you know it! The light, slightly nutty taste is a favorite for all ages.

1 bunch curly kale

3 tablespoons extra-virgin olive oil

½ teaspoon sea salt

Preheat the oven to 400°F. Line a rimmed baking sheet with aluminum foil.

Tear the kale leaves from their stems into roughly 2-inch pieces. Wash the kale and pat dry with a paper towel. Spread out the kale on the baking sheet. Drizzle with the oil and sprinkle on ¼ teaspoon of the salt. Using your hands, toss the kale, rubbing the oil into the leaves so they are fully coated. Spread the kale out so that the pieces are not overlapping too much (use a second baking sheet if necessary).

Bake the kale for 12 to 15 minutes, or until crispy. Once the chips are done, sprinkle on the remaining ¼ teaspoon salt.

Sweet and Savory Granola

Prep time: 10 minutes
Cook time: 18 minutes
Serves 4

This light, crunchy granola is incredibly simple to make and is great for breakfast, as a snack, or to satisfy a sweet or salt craving! While

I suggest using pumpkin seeds or chopped pecans here, feel free to improvise with any nuts or seeds you have on hand. You can also add shredded coconut, hemp seeds, flaxseed, or your favorite dried fruit.

2 cups quick oats

3 tablespoons oat flour (quick oats ground in a blender or food processor) or whole-wheat flour

1 teaspoon ground cinnamon

¼ teaspoon coarse sea salt

⅓ cup extra-virgin olive oil

⅓ cup pure maple syrup

⅓ cup raw pumpkin seeds or chopped raw pecans

⅓ cup raisins or dried cranberries

Preheat the oven to 350°F. Line a rimmed baking sheet with parchment paper.

In a large bowl, whisk together the oats, flour, cinnamon, and salt. Add the oil, maple syrup, pumpkin seeds, and raisins and mix until incorporated. Pour the granola onto the baking sheet and spread into a ½-inch layer.

Bake the granola for 18 minutes, or until lightly browned on top. Set aside to fully cool. Break up the granola slightly so that it is crumbly, with some larger pieces intact.

Chocolate Power Balls

Prep time: 10 minutes
Serves 4

A great fix for a sweet tooth, a midday energy slump, or a snack on the go, these treats are gluten-free and egg-free. Kids love them, and they're easy to throw together in a snap. Want to cut out the chocolate chips? Try chopped dates or dried cranberries instead.

- 1 cup quick oats
- ¼ cup natural peanut butter
- 3 to 4 tablespoons plain unsweetened almond milk or low-fat milk
- 2 tablespoons pure maple syrup
- 2 tablespoons ground flaxseed
- 1½ tablespoons unsweetened cocoa powder
- 1 teaspoon ground cinnamon
- ¼ teaspoon sea salt
- ¼ cup mini semisweet chocolate chips

In a medium bowl, combine the oats, peanut butter, 3 tablespoons of the milk, the maple syrup, flaxseed, cocoa powder, cinnamon, and salt. Mix until the ingredients are well combined, adding up to 1 tablespoon additional milk if needed. Mix in the chocolate chips. Scoop the batter using a tablespoon and roll into balls. Store the balls in an airtight container in the refrigerator.

Gingerbread Mousse with Blackberries

Prep time: 10 minutes, plus 30 minutes to chill
Serves 5

This recipe uses Greek yogurt and rich cashew butter to mimic the velvety texture of traditional buttery mousse. It's sweetened with pure maple syrup and molasses, not refined sugar. We use blackberries, but you could use strawberries or raspberries as well.

243

2 cups low-fat plain Greek yogurt

½ cup cashew butter

⅓ cup pure maple syrup

1½ teaspoons fancy molasses

½ teaspoon ground cinnamon

¼ teaspoon ground ginger

Pinch ground cloves

1 cup blackberries

In a large bowl, combine the yogurt and cashew butter. Using a hand mixer on low, mix for 2 minutes, or until smooth and creamy (or whisk by hand). Add the maple syrup, molasses, cinnamon, ginger, and cloves and mix for another 2 minutes. Divide evenly among five serving bowls. Place in the refrigerator for 30 minutes. Top each bowl with a few blackberries before serving.

Apple Quinoa Muffins

Prep time: 15 minutes
Cook time: 20 minutes
Serves 12

For the perfect snack—pre-workout or on the go—try these muffins. They're loaded with fiber and are made from simple ingredients found in your pantry.

½ cup quinoa, rinsed

1 cup water

1¾ cups spelt flour or whole-wheat flour

¼ cup unrefined sugar

1 teaspoon baking soda

1 teaspoon baking powder

1 teaspoon ground cinnamon

1 teaspoon ground ginger

¼ teaspoon sea salt

2 apples, cored and grated (unpeeled)

1 large egg, beaten

⅓ cup sunflower oil

¼ cup pure maple syrup

½ cup semisweet chocolate chips

In a medium saucepan, combine the quinoa and water and bring to a boil over high heat. Reduce the heat to low, cover, and cook for 15 to 20 minutes, or until light and fluffy. Let cool.

Preheat the oven to 350°F. Lightly grease or spray a muffin tin with olive oil.

In a large bowl, whisk together the flour, sugar, baking soda, baking powder, cinnamon, ginger, and salt. Add the cooled quinoa, apples, egg, oil, and maple syrup and mix. Gently fold in the chocolate chips. Using a ¼-cup measure, scoop the batter into the muffin cups.

Bake for 18 to 20 minutes, or until an inserted toothpick comes out clean.

Grilled Pink Grapefruit with Walnuts

Prep time: 10 minutes
Cook time: 5 minutes
Serves 4

Your friends and family will applaud you for this beautiful dessert — and they don't need to know how simple it is to prepare! You can serve it with vanilla Greek yogurt instead of ice cream for an even lighter version.

    2 large pink grapefruits

    1 teaspoon extra-virgin olive oil

    ¼ teaspoon sea salt

    4 scoops coconut ice cream or vanilla frozen yogurt

    ⅓ cup whole raw walnuts

Slice off the top and bottom of each grapefruit, then cut off the peel. Be sure to remove all the white pith. Cut into ½-inch-thick rounds. Remove any seeds.

Heat a grill pan or sauté pan over medium-high heat. Put the grapefruit slices in the pan and cook them for 2 minutes on each side, or until they're caramelized and golden brown. Arrange the slices on a plate. Drizzle the oil over them and sprinkle on the salt. Top with ice cream and walnuts.

Pumpkin Chocolate Chip Cookies

Prep time: 15 minutes
Cook time: 12 minutes
Serves 8

What a delicious way to get a little pumpkin into your diet! Pumpkin is an excellent source of beta-carotene, a powerful antioxidant that helps prevent certain types of cancers and preserves brain health. It is also loaded with potassium and zinc, and is high in fiber. Feel free to substitute raisins, currants, or dried cranberries for the chocolate chips.

    ¾ cup canned pumpkin puree (not pumpkin pie filling)

    ⅓ cup vegetable-based soft margarine

¼ cup pure maple syrup

1 large egg, beaten

1 teaspoon pure vanilla extract

¼ cup unrefined sugar

2 cups spelt flour or whole-wheat flour

½ teaspoon baking soda

½ teaspoon sea salt

1½ teaspoons ground cinnamon

¼ teaspoon ground nutmeg

¼ teaspoon ground cloves

⅓ cup semisweet chocolate chips

Preheat the oven to 375°F. Line a rimmed baking sheet with parchment paper.

In a large bowl, mix the pumpkin, margarine, maple syrup, egg, vanilla, and sugar until smooth. Add the flour, baking soda, salt, cinnamon, nutmeg, and cloves and mix until combined. Fold in the chocolate chips. Spoon the dough onto the baking sheet in mounds the size of golf balls.

Bake for 12 minutes, or until the edges are slightly golden.

Decadent Brownie Bites

Prep time: 15 minutes, plus 30 minutes to chill
Cook time: 15 minutes
Serves 8

These brownies are unbelievably rich, and yet they don't contain flour, butter, or sugar. Make them for a party or for yourself! They freeze well. I recommend using Medjool dates, which are sticky and soft; if you can only find harder dates, try soaking them in warm water before using them.

3 cups finely chopped Medjool dates

⅓ cup plain unsweetened almond milk or low-fat milk

¼ cup unsweetened cocoa powder

1 teaspoon pure vanilla extract

¼ teaspoon sea salt

1 cup chopped raw walnuts

1 cup thinly sliced strawberries

Preheat the oven to 350°F. Lightly grease or spray an 8-inch square baking pan with olive oil.

In a large bowl, combine the dates, milk, cocoa powder, vanilla, and salt. Mix until it's mostly smooth. Gently fold in the walnuts. The batter will be thick and gooey. Transfer the mixture to the baking pan and press it down with damp hands until it is evenly distributed.

Bake for 15 minutes. Set aside to cool a bit, then place the pan in the refrigerator for 30 minutes. Cut five rows each way to make 25 brownie bites. Top each brownie with a strawberry slice.

Warm Blueberry Crisp

Prep time: 12 minutes
Cook time: 30 minutes
Serves 6

We love a simple blueberry crisp for its brain-enhancing nutrients. This version uses coconut oil instead of butter for a higher dose of healthy fats. Serve on its own or with coconut ice cream or frozen yogurt.

1½ cups quick oats

¾ cup spelt flour or whole-wheat flour

2 tablespoons unrefined sugar

1 teaspoon ground cinnamon

¼ teaspoon ground nutmeg

½ cup pure maple syrup

⅓ cup coconut oil

Grated zest and juice of 1 lemon

2 tablespoons honey

5 cups blueberries

Preheat the oven to 350°F.

In a medium bowl, whisk together the oats, flour, sugar, cinnamon, and nutmeg. Add the maple syrup and coconut oil and combine until it's in pea-size pieces. (If the coconut oil is solid, use your hands.)

In a medium bowl, whisk together the lemon zest, lemon juice, and honey. Add the blueberries and toss to coat. Transfer the blueberries to an 8-inch square baking pan. Top the berries with the crumble mixture to evenly coat.

Bake the crisp for 25 to 30 minutes, or until golden brown and bubbly.

Acknowledgments

This work is a culmination of the influences of so many people over the course of my career. I had the benefit of mentors at the top of their fields in nutrition, including Walter Willett and Frank Sacks, and aging, including Denis Evans, Robert Wallace, and Frank Kohout. I developed a strong foundation in nutrition and epidemiology through endless discussions with my fellow doctoral students at the Harvard T.H. Chan School of Public Health: Susan Hankinson, Catherine Hayes, Murray Mittleman, Eric Rimm, Seth Wells, Michelle Williams, Francine Grodstein, Ed Giovanucci, and Alberto Ascherio. I am particularly grateful to the wonderful multidisciplinary team at Rush University that I've worked with for most of my career to develop the cohort studies that led to so many discoveries about nutrition, aging, and dementia. Specifically, I'd like to acknowledge Denis Evans, Julie Schneider, Christy Tangney, David Bennett, Robert Wilson, Laurel Beckett, Julia Bienias, Liesi Hebert, Paul Scherr, Judy McCann, Neelum Aggarwal, Lisa Barnes, Carlos Mendes de Leon, and David Gilley. Dallas Anderson and Laurie Ryan of the National Institute on Aging provided much-appreciated support and guidance in the pursuit and execution of my research grants to explore nutrition and dementia.

Many thanks to our agents, John Maas and Celeste Fine, for their tireless efforts on behalf of the production of this book, and to my son, Patrick who supplied invaluable legal and practical insight. Our editor, Tracy Behar, not only provided great advice on the writing, but also kept us energized and encouraged all the way to the final draft. We are also thankful for the layman's touch provided by Kristina Grish, and for Kristen Mendiola's beautiful photographs of Laura's recipes, so artfully styled by Sherrie Tan.

My children, Clare, Laura, and Patrick, inspired me to study nutrition and health in the first place, and throughout their lives they have been incredibly supportive and patient with their nerdy mother's science career, for which I am forever grateful. My two biggest supporters by far, and the foundation that allowed me to pursue my research passions, were my mother and my dear late husband, Jim. They were the keys to my research accomplishments that informed this work.

—*Dr. Martha Clare Morris*

I would like to acknowledge the culinary instructors at Northwest Culinary Academy, particularly Chef Tony Minichiello, whose enthusiasm and encouragement of nutritious culinary exploration sparked my confidence in the kitchen. I am forever grateful to Dr. Christy Tangney, whose mentorship and love of nutrition and dietary counseling guided my journey into teaching healthy living.

Many thanks to the magnificent Maureen Wilson of Sweat Co. workout studios and all the brilliant trainers there who inspire me to be a better person and personal trainer every day.

I must thank my clients—past, present, and future—for putting your health and trust in my hands. You inspire, motivate, and teach me as you go along your own journeys.

Thanks also to my wonderful friend Ashley Alexander, who

helped me transcribe recipes and kept me on track throughout this process.

I would like to thank my husband, Dr. Darcy Marr, who not only helped me organize my thoughts and ideas, taste-tested endless recipes, and took care of our small children while I was busy creating, but also offered his extensive expertise on the body and mind. I would be lost without his never-ending patience and love.

Most important, I would like to thank my mother, Dr. Martha Clare Morris, for believing in me and guiding me through this process. Her relentless passion for life and finding the truth makes me a better person every day.

—*Laura Morris*

Notes

1. Schneider JA, Arvanitakis Z, Bang W, Bennett DA. Mixed brain pathologies account for most dementia cases in community-dwelling older persons.
   Neurology 2007 Dec 11;69:2197-2204.
2. Sperling RA, Aisen PS, Beckett LA, et al. Toward defining the preclinical
   stages of Alzheimer's disease: recommendations from the National Institute
   on Aging-Alzheimer's Association workgroups on diagnostic guidelines for
   Alzheimer's disease. *Alzheimers Dement* 2011 May;7:280-292.
3. Knowler WC, Barrett-Connor E, Fowler SE, et al. Reduction in the incidence of type 2 diabetes with lifestyle intervention or metformin. *N Engl
   J Med* 2002 Feb 7;346:393-403.
4. Ngandu T, Lehtisalo J, Solomon A, et al. A 2 year multidomain intervention of diet, exercise, cognitive training, and vascular risk monitoring versus control to prevent cognitive decline in at-risk elderly people (FINGER):
   a randomised controlled trial. *Lancet* 2015 Mar 11;385:2255-2263.
5. Hendrie HC, Ogunniyi A, Hall KS, et al. Incidence of dementia and
   Alzheimer disease in 2 communities: Yoruba residing in Ibadan, Nigeria,
   and African Americans residing in Indianapolis, Indiana. *JAMA* 2001 Feb
   14;285:739-747.
6. Colcombe SJ, Erickson KI, Scalf PE, et al. Aerobic exercise training
   increases brain volume in aging humans. *J Gerontol A Biol Sci Med Sci* 2006
   Nov;61:1166-1170.
7. James BD, Wilson RS, Barnes LL, Bennett DA. Late-life social activity and
   cognitive decline in old age. *J Int Neuropsychol Soc* 2011 Nov;17:998-1005.
8. Wilson RS, Boyle PA, James BD, Leurgans SE, Buchman AS, Bennett DA.
   Negative social interactions and risk of mild cognitive impairment in old
   age. *Neuropsychology* 2015 Jul;29:561-570.
9. Wilson RS, Krueger KR, Arnold SE, et al. Loneliness and risk of Alzheimer
   disease. *Arch Gen Psychiatry* 2007 Feb;64:234-240.
10. Wilson RS, Evans DA, Bienias JL, Mendes De Leon CF, Schneider JA,

Bennett DA. Proneness to psychological distress is associated with risk of Alzheimer's disease. *Neurology* 2003 Dec 9;61:1479-1485.

11. Boyle PA, Buchman AS, Wilson RS, Yu L, Schneider JA, Bennett DA. Effect of purpose in life on the relation between Alzheimer disease pathologic changes on cognitive function in advanced age. *Arch Gen Psychiatry* 2012 May;69:499-505.

12. Grodstein F, Kang JH, Glynn RJ, Cook NR, Gaziano JM. A randomized trial of beta carotene supplementation and cognitive function in men: the Physicians' Health Study II. *Arch Intern Med* 2007 Nov 12;167:2184-2190.

13. Feart C, Letenneur L, Helmer C, Samieri C, Schalch W, Etheve S, et al. Plasma carotenoids are inversely associated with dementia risk in an elderly French cohort. *J Gerontol A Biol Sci Med Sci* 2016 May;71:683-688.

14. Morris MC, Evans DA, Bienias JL, et al. Dietary fats and the risk of incident Alzheimer's disease. *Arch Neurol* 2003;60:194-200.

15. Morris MC, Evans DA, Bienias JL, Tangney CC, Wilson RS. Dietary fat intake and 6-year cognitive change in an older biracial community population. *Neurology* 2004 May 11;62:1573-1579.

16. Estruch R, Ros E, Salas-Salvado J, et al. Primary prevention of cardiovascular disease with a Mediterranean diet. *N Engl J Med* 2013 Apr 4;368:1279-1290.

17. Vellas B, Coley N, Ousset PJ, et al. Long-term use of standardised ginkgo biloba extract for the prevention of Alzheimer's disease (GuidAge): a randomised placebo-controlled trial. *Lancet Neurol* 2012 Oct;11:851-859.

18. DeKosky ST, Williamson JD, Fitzpatrick AL, et al. Ginkgo biloba for prevention of dementia: a randomized controlled trial. *JAMA* 2008 Nov 19;300:2253-2262.

19. Snitz BE, O'Meara ES, Carlson MC, et al. Ginkgo biloba for preventing cognitive decline in older adults: a randomized trial. *JAMA* 2009 Dec 23;302:2663-2670.

20. Sano M, Ernesto C, Thomas RG, et al. A controlled trial of selegiline, alpha-tocopherol, or both as treatment for Alzheimer's disease. *N Engl J Med* 1997 Apr;336:1216-1222.

21. Dysken MW, Sano M, Asthana S, Vertrees JE, Pallaki M, Llorente M, et al. Effect of vitamin E and memantine on functional decline in Alzheimer disease: the TEAM-AD VA cooperative randomized trial. *JAMA* 2014 Jan 1;311:33-44.

22. Petersen RC, Thomas RG, Grundman M, et al. Vitamin E and donepezil for the treatment of mild cognitive impairment. *N Engl J Med* 2005 Jun 9;352:2379-2388.

23. Kang JH, Cook NR, Manson JE, Buring JE, Albert CM, Grodstein F. Vitamin E, vitamin C, beta carotene, and cognitive function among women with or at risk of cardiovascular disease. *Circulation* 2009 Jun 2;119:2772-2780.

24. Kang JH, Cook N, Manson J, Buring JE, Grodstein F. A randomized trial of vitamin E supplementation and cognitive function in women. *Arch Intern Med* 2006 Dec 11;166:2462-2468.

25. Kang JH, Ascherio A, Grodstein F. Fruit and vegetable consumption and cognitive decline in aging women. *Ann Neurol* 2005 May;57:713-720.

26. Nooyens AC, Bueno-de-Mesquita HB, van Boxtel MP, van Gelder BM, Verhagen H, Verschuren WM. Fruit and vegetable intake and cognitive decline in middle-aged men and women: the Doetinchem Cohort Study. *Br J Nutr* 2011 Sep;106:752-761.

27. Morris MC, Evans DA, Tangney CC, Bienias JL, Wilson RS. Associations of vegetable and fruit consumption with age-related cognitive change. *Neurology* 2006 Oct 24;67:1370-1376.

28. Mozaffarian D, Hao T, Rimm EB, Willett WC, Hu FB. Changes in diet and lifestyle and long-term weight gain in women and men. *N Engl J Med* 2011 June;364:2392-4204.

29. Muraki I, Rimm E, Willett WC, Manson JE, Hu FB, Sun Q. Potato consumption and risk of type 2 diabetes: results from three prospective cohort studies. *Diabetes Care* 2016 Mar;39:376-384.

30. Borgi L, Rimm EB, Willett WC, Forman JP. Potato intake and incidence of hypertension: results from three prospective US cohort studies. *BMJ* 2016 May17;353:i2351.

31. Mozaffarian RS, Lee RM, Kennedy MA, Ludwig DS, Mozaffarian D, Gortmaker SL. Identifying whole grain foods: a comparison of different approaches for selecting more healthful whole grain products. *Public Health Nutr* 2013 Dec;16:2255-2264.

32. Martinez-Lapiscina EH, Clavero P, Toledo E, et al. Mediterranean diet improves cognition: the PREDIMED-NAVARRA randomised trial. *J Neurol Neurosurg Psychiatry* 2013 Dec;84:1318-1325.

33. Casas R, Sacanella E, Urpí-Sardà M, Corella D, Castañer O, Lamuela-Raventos RM, et al. Long-term immunomodulatory effects of a Mediterranean diet in adults at high risk of cardiovascular disease in the PREvención con DIeta MEDiterránea (PREDIMED) randomized controlled trial. *J Nutr* 2016 Sep;146:1684-1693.

34. Shukitt-Hale B, Bielinski DF, Lau FC, Willis LM, Carey AN, Joseph JA. The beneficial effects of berries on cognition, motor behaviour and neuronal function in ageing. *Br J Nutr* 2015 Nov 28;114:1542-1549.

35. Devore EE, Kang JH, Breteler MM, Grodstein F. Dietary intakes of berries and flavonoids in relation to cognitive decline. *Ann Neurol* 2012 Jul;72:135-143.

36. Samieri C, Sun Q, Townsend MK, Rimm EB, Grodstein F. Dietary flavonoid intake at midlife and healthy aging in women. *Am J Clin Nutr* 2014 Dec;100:1489-1497.

37. Miller MG, Hamilton DA, Joseph JA, Shukitt-Hale B. Dietary blueberry improves cognition among older adults in a randomized, double-blind, placebo-controlled trial. *Eur J Nutr* 2017 Mar;10:1-12.

38. Willis LM, Shukitt-Hale B, Cheng V, Joseph JA. Dose-dependent effects of walnuts on motor and cognitive function in aged rats. *Br J Nutr* 2009 Apr;101:1140-1144.

39. Mastroiacovo D, Kwik-Uribe C, Grassi D, Necozione S, Raffaele A, Pistacchio L, et al. Cocoa flavanol consumption improves cognitive function, blood pressure control, and metabolic profile in elderly subjects: the Cocoa, Cognition, and Aging (CoCoA) Study—a randomized controlled trial. *Am J Clin Nutr* 2015 Mar;101:538-548.

40. Albanese E, Dangour AD, Uauy R, et al. Dietary fish and meat intake and dementia in Latin America, China, and India: a 10/66 Dementia Research Group population-based study. *Am J Clin Nutr* 2009 Aug;90:392-400.

41. Morris MC, Brockman J, Schneider JA, et al. Association of seafood consumption, brain mercury level, and APOE ε4 status with brain neuropathology in older adults. *JAMA* 2016 Feb 2;315:489-497.

42. van de Rest O, Wang Y, Barnes LL, Tangney C, Bennett DA, Morris MC. APOE ε4 and the associations of seafood and long-chain omega-3 fatty acids with cognitive decline. *Neurology* 2016 May 31;86:2063-2070.

43. Gerstenberger SL, Martinson A, Kramer JL. An evaluation of mercury concentrations in three brands of canned tuna. *Environ Toxicol Chem* 2010 Feb;29:237-242.

44. Morris MC, Evans DA, Bienias JL, et al. Dietary niacin and risk of incident Alzheimer's disease and of cognitive decline. *J Neurol Neurosurg Psych* 2004 Aug;75:1093-1099.

45. Morris MC, Evans DA, Bienias JL, et al. Dietary fats and the risk of incident Alzheimer's disease. *Arch Neurol* 2003;60:194-200.

46. Cahill LE, Pan A, Chiuve SE, et al. Fried-food consumption and risk of type 2 diabetes and coronary artery disease: a prospective study in 2 cohorts of US women and men. *Am J Clin Nutr* 2014 Aug;100:667-675.

47. Yang Q, Zhang Z, Gregg EW, Flanders WD, Merritt R, Hu FB. Added sugar intake and cardiovascular diseases mortality among US adults. *JAMA Intern Med* 2014 Apr;174:516-524.

48. Soar K, Chapman E, Lavan N, Jansari A, Turner J. Investigating the effects of caffeine on executive functions using traditional Stroop and a new ecologically-valid virtual reality task, the Jansari assessment of Executive Functions (JEF(©)). *Appetite* 2016 Oct;105:156-163.

49. Urribarri J, Woodruff S, Goodwin S, Cai W, Chen X, et al. Advanced glycation end products in foods and a practical guide to their reduction in the diet. *J Am Diet Assoc* 2010 Jun;110:911-916.

50. Keys A. Seven countries: a multivariate analysis of death and coronary heart disease. Cambridge, MA: Harvard University Press, 1980.

51. Lopez-Garcia E, Rodriguez-Artalejo F, Li TY, et al. The Mediterranean-style dietary pattern and mortality among men and women with cardio-vascular disease. *Am J Clin Nutr* 2014 Jan;99:172-180.

52. Scarmeas N, Stern Y, Tang MX, Mayeux R, Luchsinger JA. Mediterranean diet and risk for Alzheimer's disease. *Ann Neurol* 2006 Jun;59:912-921.

53. Appel LJ, Moore TJ, Obarzanek E, et al. A clinical trial of the effects of dietary patterns on blood pressure. DASH Collaborative Research Group. *New Engl J Med* 1997 Apr;336:1117-1124.

54. Smith PJ, Blumenthal JA, Babyak MA, Craighead L, Welsh-Bohmer KA, Browndyke JN, Strauman TA, Sherwood A. Effects of the dietary approaches to stop hypertension diet, exercise, and caloric restriction on neuro-cognition in overweight adults with high blood pressure. *Hypertension* 2010 Jun;55:1331-1338.

55. Morris MC, Tangney CC, Wang Y, Sacks FM, Bennett DA, Aggarwal NT. MIND diet associated with reduced incidence of Alzheimer's disease. *Alzheimers Dement* 2015 Sep;11:1007-1014.

56. Morris MC, Tangney CC, Wang Y, et al. MIND diet slows cognitive decline with aging. *Alzheimers Dement* 2015 Sep;11:1015-1022.

Index

About the Authors

Dr. Martha Clare Morris is a professor of epidemiology, director of the Rush Institute on Healthy Aging in the Department of Internal Medicine, and assistant provost of Community Research at Rush University Medical Center in Chicago. She received her doctoral degree in epidemiology from the Harvard T.H. Chan School of Public Health. She has more than twenty years of experience studying risk factors in the development of Alzheimer's disease and other health problems of older people, and in particular how nutrition relates to these conditions. Dr. Morris has published findings on the relationships of dietary patterns, antioxidant nutrients, dietary fats, and the B vitamins to these conditions. She is the lead creator of the MIND diet for healthy brain aging. She has a long history of NIH and other funding to examine dietary risk factors of Alzheimer's disease among 10,000 African American and Caucasian participants of the Chicago Health and Aging Project, as well as the relationship of diet and brain metals to neuropathology and neurologic diseases among 1,200 Chicago participants of the Memory and Aging Project. She is also the principal investigator of a multicenter randomized trial of the MIND diet to prevent Alzheimer's disease. Dr. Morris lives in Chicago. She has three children, Clare, Laura, and Patrick, and four grandchildren, Nolan, Kelly, Maxwell, and Colin.

Dr. Morris's daughter, Laura Morris, is a certified personal trainer, certified nutrition consultant, and professionally trained chef. Laura has experience working with a variety of age groups and special populations, including elite athletes, cancer patients, busy working professionals, and even public personalities. Laura's passions for fitness and nutrition were cultivated at an early age. She has gained both experience and knowledge working in the clinical nutrition department at Rush University Medical Center in Chicago. Laura's culinary arts education has allowed her to better apply her knowledge of nutrition to food preparation and diet execution. Laura is always seeking ways to assist her clients as they find their path to eating, exercising, and living their best. She lives and works in Vancouver, British Columbia, with her husband, Darcy Marr, and their kids, Nolan and Kelly.